T5-BBA-498

NEW DIRECTIONS FOR MENTAL HEALTH SERVICES

H. Richard Lamb, *University of Southern California*
EDITOR-IN-CHIEF

Effective Psychiatric Rehabilitation

Robert Paul Liberman
UCLA School of Medicine

EDITOR

Number 53, Spring 1992

JOSSEY-BASS PUBLISHERS
San Francisco

EFFECTIVE PSYCHIATRIC REHABILITATION
Robert Paul Liberman (ed.)
New Directions for Mental Health Services, no. 53
H. Richard Lamb, Editor-in-Chief

Microfilm copies of issues and articles are available in 16mm and 35mm,
as well as microfiche in 105mm, through University Microfilms Inc., 300
North Zeeb Road, Ann Arbor, Michigan 48106.

LC 87-646993   ISSN 0193-9416   ISBN 1-55542-757-X

NEW DIRECTIONS FOR MENTAL HEALTH SERVICES is part of The Jossey-
Bass Social and Behavioral Sciences Series and is published quarterly by
Jossey-Bass Publishers, 350 Sansome Street, San Francisco, California
94104-1310 (publication number USPS 493-910). Second-class postage
paid at San Francisco, California, and at additional mailing offices.
POSTMASTER: Send address changes to New Directions for Mental Health
Services, Jossey-Bass Publishers, 350 Sansome Street, San Francisco, Cal-
ifornia 94104-1310.

SUBSCRIPTIONS for 1992 cost $48.00 for individuals and $70.00 for institutions, agencies, and libraries.

EDITORIAL CORRESPONDENCE should be sent to the Editor-in-Chief,
H. Richard Lamb, Department of Psychiatry and the Behavioral Sciences,
U.S.C. School of Medicine, 1934 Hospital Place, Los Angeles, California
90033.

Cover photograph by Wernher Krutein/PHOTOVAULT © 1990.

Printed on acid-free paper in the United States of America.

CONTENTS

EDITOR'S NOTES   1
Robert Paul Liberman

1. Assessment and Treatment of Cognitive Impairments   7
Dorie Reed, Mary E. Sullivan, David L. Penn, Paul Stuve,
William D. Spaulding
Impairments in cognitive functioning, which obstruct psychiatric rehabili-
tation, are resistant to drugs and conventional psychosocial treatment but
can be reduced by specialized training techniques.

2. A Cognitive-Behavioral Treatment Program for Patients with   21
a Schizophrenic Disorder
Carlo Perris
The multidetermined nature of the disability of patients suffering from
schizophrenic disorders requires a comprehensive treatment approach that
includes cognitive-behavioral therapy.

3. Combining Social Skills Training and Assertive Case   33
Management: The Social and Independent Living Skills Program
of the Brentwood Veterans Affairs Medical Center
Jerome V. Vaccaro, Robert P. Liberman, Charles J. Wallace, Gayla Blackwell
A clinical research program for persons suffering from schizophrenia has
been designed to optimize the additive effects of social skills training and
assertive case management.

4. Family-Aided Assertive Community Treatment: 43
A Comprehensive Rehabilitation and Intensive Case Management
Approach for Persons with Schizophrenic Disorders
William R. McFarlane, Peter Stastny, Susan Deakins
By combining the therapeutic and rehabilitative effects of assertive community treatment, family psychoeducation, and the multifamily group, better
use of an expanded social network yields a more coordinated clinical effort
and an enhanced level of community adaptation for patients with chronic
schizophrenia.

5. Effectively Treating Stimulant-Abusing Schizophrenics: 55
Mission Impossible?
Lisa J. Roberts, Andrew Shaner, Thad A. Eckman,
Douglas E. Tucker, Jerome V. Vaccaro
Rehabilitation of individuals with concomitant schizophrenia and stimulant
abuse, once deemed futile, now seems feasible and promising.

6. Optimal Drug and Behavior Therapy for Treatment-Refractory   67
Institutionalized Schizophrenics
Timothy G. Kuehnel, Robert P. Liberman,
Barringer D. Marshall, Jr., Linda Bowen
Institutionalized persons with a deteriorating form of schizophrenia that
was refractory to neuroleptic medication were titrated downward in their
haloperidol dose. Based on ratings of their clinical status, an optimal dose
was reached that was an average 66 percent reduction from their initial
levels. Patients then participated in a personalized, intensive behavior therapy program to remediate their extreme, persisting deficits and disturbances in behavior.

7. Ecological Vocational Rehabilitation   79
J. P. Dauwalder, H. Hoffmann
Chronicity in serious mental disorders emanates from deficient ecological
resources interacting with vulnerable individuals. Rehabilitation can succeed if an integrated and individualized approach is augmented by appropriate ecological supports.

8. Choose-Get-Keep: A Psychiatric Rehabilitation Approach to   87
Supported Employment
Karen S. Danley, Ken Sciarappa, Kim MacDonald-Wilson
By implementing intervention strategies to help psychiatrically disabled
persons choose, get, and keep jobs, supported employment can become a
successful element in psychiatric rehabilitation.

9. The Growth of Supported Employment from Horticulture   97
Therapy in the Veterans' Garden
Jerome V. Vaccaro, Ida Cousino, Robert Vatcher
While institution-bound programs in horticulture therapy were appropriate
for the era in which long-term hospitalization was the primary mode of
psychiatric treatment, the supported employment paradigm updates this
mode of treatment for the current era of community psychiatry.

10. The Job-Finding Module: Training Skills for Seeking   105
Competitive Community Employment
Harvey E. Jacobs, Rosemary Collier, Donald Wissusik
Developed from eight years of research, the Job-Finding Module is designed
to help persons with disabilities who are capable of returning to the work
force obtain competitive community employment.

INDEX   117

EDITOR'S NOTES

With well-replicated, international studies showing that half or more of persons diagnosed as having schizophrenia experience substantial social and symptomatic recoveries twenty to thirty years after their florid illnesses began (Ciompi, 1980; Huber, Gross, Schuttler, and Gross, 1980; Harding, Brooks, Ashikaga, and Strauss, 1987; Liberman, 1988), the question is no longer whether or not schizophrenia and related serious mental disorders are treatable but rather what can be done to accelerate functional recoveries in such individuals. The framework of "vulnerability-stress-protective" factors for understanding the course and outcome of serious mental disorders, depicted in Figure 1, provides a map for directing treatment and rehabilitation strategies for the seriously mentally ill, the operational premise being that early intervention more rapidly reduces impairments, disabilities, and handicaps associated with mental illnesses (Mueser, Liberman, and Glynn, 1990).

Positive and negative symptoms of schizophrenia and their associated social and personal disabilities are the consequences of stress impinging on an individual's enduring psychobiological vulnerability to schizophrenic disorder. This vulnerability is thought to be determined by genetic loading, putative neurotransmitter dysfunctions, and structural or lesional brain abnormalities, and it may result in cognitive, autonomic, or attentional impairments. Coping skills enable the individual to reduce or adapt successfully to environmental stress and hence modulate the noxious effects of stress on vulnerability. Evidence abounds that premorbid and postmorbid social competence and coping skills contribute to adequate social adjustment and are predictive of a favorable outcome of the illness. According to this model, the functioning of a schizophrenic patient is reflected by the dynamic balance of protective factors (coping skill, antipsychotic medication, social support), on the one hand, and stress and vulnerability, on the other.

The role of protective factors in mitigating the impact of stressors on vulnerability has broad implications for psychosocial interventions. The interaction of coping skills, social support, stress, and vulnerability clearly identifies the therapeutic objectives of and modalities for interventions. Neuroleptic drugs can be prescribed to lessen vulnerability and to buffer the effects of stress. Environmental modification can ameliorate the noxious effects of stress on the individual by reducing the power of the stressors. Stress reduction may in part account for the benefit of hospitalization, whereby the patient is temporarily removed from stressors in the family and community. Structured, community-based, aftercare environments, such as day treatment programs, social clubs, and sheltered workshops, can be

Figure 1. Factors Affecting Mental Disorders

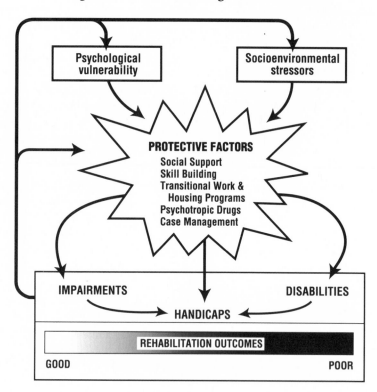

effective in providing patients with support to compensate for deficits in community living skills and with opportunities for improving the quality of their interactions with others. In addition, interventions such as case management, social skills training, and family therapy can further strengthen social support networks and improve patients' skills at coping with a range of stressors.

This volume, *Effective Psychiatric Rehabilitation,* illuminates new approaches to psychiatric rehabilitation that confer protection to individuals with a psychobiological vulnerability to socioenvironmental stressors. At the present time, our tools are insufficiently sensitive for isolating the critical neurochemical and physiological events in the brain that are responsible for the enduring vulnerability of individuals to the symptoms and disabilities of schizophrenia and other chronic disorders; thus, we cannot intervene directly with the causative, pathogenetic factors in the central nervous system. Nor can we retreat to an era of treatment where patients were given asylum for years, protected from the stressors of community life. Our contemporary ethos and priorities dictate community-based treatment and the equipping of vulnerable individuals with skills to cope with the inevitable stressors of daily living, for example, street drugs and alcohol, homelessness, interpersonal conflict, social stimulation, and stigma. Therefore, our treatment and rehabilitation efforts must entail well-designed interventions derived from pharmacotherapy, skills training, and social support.

Based on work conducted at the University of Nebraska and the Lincoln Regional Center, Dorie Reed and her colleagues, in Chapter One, describe techniques for assessing and directly remediating cognitive impairments that reflect the core psychobiological deficits and vulnerability of persons with schizophrenia. While still in the preliminary stages of development and validation, their results from a series of case studies constitute a promising counterargument to the therapeutic nihilism of biological determinism in contemporary psychiatry. It is clear from the case studies cited by Reed and her co-authors that even the cognitive and attentional deficits linked to presumed neurobiological pathology can be improved and even normalized through specialized training and motivational methods.

A multimodal approach to the treatment and rehabilitation of young adults with schizophrenia and other serious mental disorders has been developed by Carlo Perris and his interdisciplinary team at the University of Umea in Sweden. In Chapter Two, Perris describes how, with small groups of patients in a homestyle environment, cognitive therapy based on the principles previously found effective in depressive and anxiety disorder is used in combination with medication, group therapy, recreational and physical therapy, and other modalities. While it is not possible to pinpoint the specific contribution of cognitive therapy in this approach, the richness and the intensity of the comprehensive rehabilitation offered by a highly trained and motivated staff warrants the envy of most public mental health programs in the United States.

In Chapter Six, Timothy G. Kuehnel, Robert P. Liberman, Barringer D. Marshall, Jr., and Linda Bowen, at the Camarillo-UCLA Clinical Research Center, describe their work with older, treatment-refractory persons with schizophrenia, whose disabilities, persisting symptoms, and behavioral disturbances require institutional care. They have found that two-thirds reductions in the doses of antipsychotic medication yield more optimal symptomatic control with significantly fewer side effects. The benefit-risk ratio for pharmacotherapy of this difficult-to-treat population appears related to a therapeutic window for plasma levels of medication, augmenting patients' responsiveness to individualized behavior therapy for their residual deficits and disturbances.

In three chapters here, the combination of skills training with case management or family management of persons with schizophrenia is described in projects conducted in state, municipal, and veterans hospitals. In Chapter Three, Jerome V. Vaccaro, Robert P. Liberman, Charles J. Wallace, and Gayla Blackwell discuss their finding that the addition of skills training to assertive, clinical case management leads to significant improvements in the quality of life of patients, as contrasted to patients receiving psychosocial occupational therapy with case management.

A novel spin-off of involving multiple family groups in the psychosocial rehabilitation of disabled relatives has been family-operated employment agencies, which have yielded better vocational outcomes for the seriously mentally ill than has assertive case management alone. In Chapter Four, William R. McFarlane, Peter Stastny, and Susan Deakins describe how family-aided community treatment appears to give relatives a constructive role in the rehabilitation of their sick family member without unduly burdening them.

In Chapter Five, Lisa J. Roberts and her colleagues at the Brentwood VA Hospital in Los Angeles describe a multimodal program for stimulant-abusing schizophrenics that employs social skills training, training in relapse prevention, the twelve-step Alcoholics Anonymous approach, peer supports, and case management. The engagement of this hitherto treatment-resistant population in the Dual Diagnosis Treatment Program thus far has been favorable and research is being conducted to determine the program's efficacy.

The dreary record of vocational rehabilitation of the mentally ill in past years is highlighted by the fact that less than 1 percent of those on Social Security pensions are ever rehabilitated, and by the fact that less than 15 percent of all hospitalized mentally ill persons ever get jobs. New initiatives in vocational rehabilitation are described in this volume, and the initial findings are promising. The transitional employment approach, pioneered by Fountain House and its congeners in psychosocial rehabilitation, is described in Chapter Seven by J. P. Dauwalder and H. Hoffmann, who have applied the approach within a community-based system of care in Bern, Switzerland. The flexible support offered to patients by the psychosocial program and its mobile case managers leads eventually to supported employment in local industries.

In Chapter Eight, Karen S. Danley, Ken Sciarappa, and Kim MacDonald-Wilson describe their "choose-get-keep" approach to supported employment at the Boston University Center for Psychiatric Rehabilitation. In line with other reports, this approach was successful for 42 percent of the participants who held jobs at the end of the first year of the program. The key tasks of social skills training, service coordination, and employer consultation, carried out by case managers or "job coaches," were found to be instrumental in supporting the employment of participants.

The evolution of vocational rehabilitation from "work therapy" to "supported employment" at the Veterans' Garden at the Brentwood VA Hospital in Los Angeles is highlighted in Chapter Nine. Jerome V. Vaccaro, Ida Cousino, and Robert Vatcher describe how horticulture therapy contained the seeds of a supported employment initiative for mentally ill veterans who "graduated" into landscape maintenance jobs at a local university.

An important element in vocational rehabilitation is training for finding a job, and the behaviorally oriented Job Club has been shown to effectively teach job-finding skills to persons with mental disabilities. Against the backdrop of research evidence indicating that 35 to 65 percent of the mentally ill can succeed in the job search enterprise with appropriate skills training, coaching, and incentives, Harvey E. Jacobs, Rosemary Collier, and Donald Wissusik describe their Job Finding Module in Chapter Ten.

The innovations in psychiatric rehabilitation described in this volume are threatened by the reduction of resources available for the seriously mentally ill as Medicaid, Medicare, and third-party reimbursements dry up and state mental health budgets face funding crises. Also jeopardizing the further validation and dissemination of effective methods of psychiatric rehabilitation are the "turf" wars now heating up between organized psychiatry and allied mental health disciplines. Unless dramatic new solutions to the organization, financing, and delivery of mental health services can be crafted, rehabilitation may be stifled at the very time that its promise is being realized.

Previous issues of New Directions for Mental Health Services have examined innovations in the organization and financing of services for the seriously mentally ill, including capitation and training in community living. One unexamined innovation is the delivery of psychiatric services through primary care practitioners, in consultation with teams of experts in psychiatric treatment and rehabilitation. With the growth of health maintenance organizations and other provider networks that have primary care practitioners as "gatekeepers" for mental health service delivery, it is conceivable that psychiatric expertise—including the provision of specialized rehabilitative services—could be organized around locally responsible and accountable primary care practitioners.

In an experiment conducted in Buckinghamshire, England, close liaison of psychiatric teams with general practitioners resulted in early detection of florid episodes of major mental disorders, rapidly responsive crisis intervention, and family-based methods of treatment and rehabilitation. The warning signs of imminent relapse were identified and employed as clinical markers of vulnerability to stress-induced exacerbations. Patients, family members, other caregivers, and general practitioners were all instructed to respond in a coordinated and efficient manner whenever such warning signs were noted. The liaison team of mental health practitioners was expertly trained in pharmacotherapy and psychosocial rehabilitation, providing these specialized services in close consultation with the primary care doctors. A pilot study of this integrated approach found a tenfold reduction in the development of new cases of chronic schizophrenia during a five-year period (Falloon, Shanahan, Krekorian, and Laporta, 1990).

Innovations in the services and programs available to the seriously mentally ill will translate to cost-effective advances in treatment and rehabilitation when organized, delivered, and financed in ways that ensure quality, consistency, continuity, and commitment to this long-underserved population. The reports of innovations in services found in this volume represent advances that can be readily used by consumers, providers, and administrators of programs for the seriously mentally ill.

Robert Paul Liberman
Editor

References

Ciompi, L. "Atamnestic Long-Term Study of the Course of Life and Aging of Schizophrenics." *Schizophrenia Bulletin*, 1980, *6*, 606–618.

Falloon, I.R.H., Shanahan, W., Krekorian, H.A.R., and Laporta, M. "Integrated Family, General Practice, and Mental Health Care in the Management of Schizophrenia." *Journal of the Royal Society of Medicine*, 1990, *83*, 225–228.

Harding, C. M., Brooks, G. W., Ashikaga, T., and Strauss, J. S. "The Vermont Longitudinal Study of Persons with Severe Mental Illness." *American Journal of Psychiatry*, 1987, *144*, 718–735.

Huber, G., Gross, C., Schuttler, R., and Gross, H. K. "Longitudinal Follow-up Studies of Schizophrenic Patients." *Schizophrenia Bulletin*, 1980, *6*, 592–605.

Liberman, R. P. *Psychiatric Rehabilitation of Chronic Mental Patients*. Washington, D.C.: American Psychiatric Press, 1988.

Mueser, T. I., Liberman, R. P., and Glynn, S. M. "Psychosocial Interventions in Schizophrenia." In A. Kales, C. N. Stefanis, and T.J.A. Talbott (eds.), *Recent Advances in Schizophrenia*. New York: Springer-Verlag, 1990.

ROBERT PAUL LIBERMAN, M.D., is professor of psychiatry at the UCLA School of Medicine, chief of the Rehabilitation Medicine Service at the Brentwood (Psychiatric) Division of the West Los Angeles VA Medical Center, and director of the UCLA Clinical Research Center for Schizophrenia and Psychiatric Rehabilitation.

Impairments in cognitive functioning, which obstruct psychiatric rehabilitation, are resistant to drugs and conventional psychosocial treatment but can be reduced by specialized training techniques.

Assessment and Treatment of Cognitive Impairments

Dorie Reed, Mary E. Sullivan, David L. Penn, Paul Stuve, William D. Spaulding

The many psychological processes involved with perception, attention, and thinking are collectively termed *cognition*. Cognition includes relatively simple processes such as identification of visual features and selective attention, as well as complex ones such as social perception and problem solving. A continuum from "molecular" cognition (simple, unitary processes) to "molar" cognition (complex processes), describes the exchange of information within a human being at varying levels of organization and complexity. Upward transmission of information, from molecular to more molar processes, typically results in the integration of perceptual or memory elements into increasingly more integrated and holistic constructions of the world. Downward transmission either modulates the activity of the more molecular processes, analogous to adjustments of the gain of an amplifier, or translates complex plans of action into specific motor responses.

Impairments in cognitive processes are considered basic to serious mental disorders such as schizophrenia and have detrimental effects at all levels of individual psychosocial functioning. For example, when patients are actively psychotic with severe disruption of neurophysiological and cognitive processes, they are generally not able to benefit from conventional forms of psychiatric rehabilitation. Cognitive impairments of varying severity often remain in the residual phase of psychotic disorders, despite optimal antipsychotic drug effects (Spohn and Strauss, 1989). Residual cognitive impairments can be significant obstacles to personal functioning and can impede efforts at psychosocial rehabilitation.

Cognitive impairments appear to play a significant role in the functioning and treatment responses of psychiatric patients undergoing rehabilitation. Among chronic, institutionalized schizophrenics, Spaulding, Penn, and Wiler (1990) found relationships among molar and molecular cognitive impairments, social skills, social behavior, and patterns of symptomatology. Changes in molecular cognitive functioning in residual schizophrenic patients have been shown to correspond to changes in their social functioning (Spaulding, in press). Deficits in vigilance and attention have been found to be related to poor responses to skills training (Kraemer, Zinner, and Moller, 1988; Bowen, 1988). The often-reported failure of schizophrenics to generalize social skills training to naturalistic settings may be due to the failure of skills trainers to address patients' cognitive impairments in their training procedures (Liberman, Nuechterlein, and Wallace, 1982).

One strategy for addressing cognitive impairments is to make skills training and other conventional rehabilitation modalities as sensitive as possible to the cognitive impairments of patients. This strategy has been successfully pursued in the development of techniques for social skills training by the Clinical Research Center for Schizophrenia and Psychiatric Rehabilitation at the University of California, Los Angeles (UCLA). Liberman, Nuechterlein, and Wallace's (1982) recommendations for amplifying the effects and durability of social skills training include the following: (1) Keep the training setting uncluttered and devoid of distracting stimuli. (2) Post graphic charts for clear and simple visual cuing of cognitive strategies. (3) Use mild censure for inappropriate responses as well as praise for appropriate responses. (4) Conduct task analysis and break down tasks into simple steps. (5) Decrease novelty by means of many repetitions before moving to new material or scenes.

The main advantage of this strategy is that it makes use of existent skills-training technology to compensate for patients' cognitive impairments. In addition, it is possible that skills training at the molar level improves cognitive functioning at the molecular level, especially if the training is intensive and long term. Its applicability is limited, however, because of the heterogeneity of patients' deficits. Even the most experienced and highly trained therapist cannot be expected to assess and compensate for every patient's unique constellation of cognitive deficits in the course of training sessions.

In this chapter, we present an alternative rehabilitation strategy, namely, techniques for assessing and directly remediating cognitive impairments in psychiatric rehabilitation. We then describe cognitive remediation techniques aimed at molecular-to-molar levels of cognitive functioning.

Vigilance and Continuous Performance

Vigilance is the ability to maintain readiness to respond to an expected signal over an extended period of time. Continuous performance is the result of vigilance, with emphasis on the response. Continuous performance tasks can be extremely simple, as in pushing a button in response to a signal tone. However, vigilance and continuous performance also underlie such complex activities as participation in skills training and social conversation. Even simple tasks of vigilance and continuous performance are disrupted in the acute phase of psychotic illnesses, with impairments persisting in the residual phase on tasks with complex signal characteristics or performance demands (Neuchterlein and Dawson, 1984; Neuchterlein, 1990).

In our study, commercially available packages of computerized tasks for exercising these skills, resembling very simple video games, were employed as a means of improving the continuous performance of fifteen chronic, institutionalized psychiatric patients. Subjects were selected on the basis of deficient performance on one or more tasks in a set of ten tasks, on which normal adults and even many psychiatric patients can perform perfectly. Each subject showed a unique pattern of deficits across the tasks that was not attributable to diagnostic differences. The subjects then practiced a subset of the tasks in thirty-minute sessions, two to three days per week, for eight weeks.

All but one of the subjects showed improvement on at least one of the ten tasks, but most showed improvement on less than one-half of the tasks that they practiced. The patterns of change were as unique as the patterns of initial impairment. There was no evidence of generalization from improvement on the vigilance tasks to improvement in an occupational therapy workshop program, in ambient social functioning, or in independent evaluations of cognitive functioning. While chronic psychiatric patients can change their levels of vigilance and continuous performance, the small amount of change and lack of generalization point to the need to include extrinsic rewards and transitional opportunities to plan and motivate the generalization of improvements to real-life situations.

A similar study recently completed by Dorie Reed more directly addressed motivational factors. The subjects were four chronic, institutionalized schizophrenic subjects who had previously been classified in a rigorous drug trial protocol as "minimal drug responders." The subjects practiced a variety of visual scanning and memory tasks, less intrinsically interesting than video games, in fifteen- to twenty-minute lessons, four times per week, for eighteen weeks. Continuous on-task behavior was reinforced with food at ten-minute intervals. All four of the subjects showed gradual improvement in continuous task performance. There was no evidence of generalization of this improvement to a concomitant skills-training group. Accuracy on the visual scanning and memory tasks was highly variable both between and within subjects and did not change over the course of the training. However, two of the subjects showed significant improvement in independently assessed cognitive functioning after the training period.

In a more naturalistic study of chronic institutionalized subjects who participated in a continuous performance task in which they sorted and collated in a sheltered workshop, informally delivered behavior therapy improved sustained performance in seven of nine patients (Spaulding, Storms, Goodrich, and Sullivan, 1986). However, no generalization or overall clinical improvement was associated with the improved vigilance.

Taken together, these three studies suggest that improvement on continuous performance tasks has at least two components. One component involves changes in molecular vigilance processes, and the other involves motivational factors. This analysis, in combination with the fact of heterogeneity of impairments within the domain of continuous performance, suggests that considerable individual assessment and treatment tailoring are necessary for significant treatment impact. Also, in view of the lack of spontaneous generalization, improvements in vigilance and continuous performance may be expected to have minimal impact on daily living skills unless cognitive remediation is aggressively integrated into a comprehensive rehabilitation program.

It is notable, however, that the subjects in these studies were selected for having gross impairments. Even within the population of chronic, institutionalized patients, they fall around the ninetieth percentile of severity of continuous performance impairment. Patients with less severe deficits may respond quite differently, if they need treatment in this domain at all. In any case, inasmuch as vigilance and continuous performance are key prerequisites to participation in skills training and related modalities, improvement in this domain may make rehabilitation accessible to some patients who would otherwise have a very poor prognosis, even if spontaneous generalization is very limited.

Distractibility

Distractibility is an impairment in the molecular range of cognition characterized by disruption of ongoing cognitive activity by irrelevant stimuli. Often it is difficult to distinguish between distractibility and vigilance impairments, as distraction directly disrupts vigilance; however, simple vigilance impairments can occur in the absence of distracting stimuli. The distinction is clearest when ongoing activity is disrupted by specifiable stimuli despite the patient's efforts to prevent it.

Distractibility, according to Pogue-Geile and Oltmanns (1980), is primarily associated with schizophrenia. In all people, distractibility is closely associated with psychophysiological arousal, and so it can also be observed in patients with anxiety and affective disorders and even among acutely agitated normal adults. For this reason, distractibility may sometimes be treated with relaxation training and related psychophysiological stress management techniques, with or without interventions aimed directly at cognition. Schizophrenic patients often have distractibility problems in the absence of extreme arousal, however.

The following case study illustrates the use of cognitive behavior therapy for reducing the impairments associated with distractibility:

> The patient was a twenty-three-year-old outpatient whose eight years of paranoid schizophrenic symptoms had been controlled sufficiently for him to attend courses at a university. However, his academic efforts were impaired by distractibility associated with short-term memory problems and ideas of reference, that is, feeling that classmates were talking about and laughing at him.
>
> An exercise was designed to improve his ability to efficiently apprehend the content of spoken information. Over the course of four therapy sessions, the therapist read aloud two to three sentence blocks from a newspaper article and asked the patient to describe in his own words the basic idea of the sentences. At the end of the article the patient was asked to summarize its theme. A tape of other readings, with pauses for summarization, was made so that he could practice this exercise at home. After one month, he reported an improved ability to follow lectures and reading assignments.
>
> To address the social components of his distractibility, the patient practiced a social apperception task, first described by Spaulding, Storms, Goodrich, and Sullivan (1986), involving repetitive generation of different story responses to thematic apperception test (TAT) cards. He found this to be a stimulating task. After a number of sessions, the therapist underscored the parallel between perceiving a particular TAT card in different ways and perceptions of actual social situations. For example, the patient was asked to generate as many different perceptions and interpretations as possible of a situation that he had automatically associated with ridicule, such as hearing other students whispering in class. The plausibility of each of the different interpretations was then discussed, with an emphasis on assessing the likelihood that particular interpretations were correct. He was then given homework assignments to practice this exercise whenever he thought that people were talking about him. This task was also practiced in vivo by going to the Student Union with the therapist and discussing alternative interpretations whenever he thought others were watching or talking about him. At the end of six months, he reported feeling less distracted by paranoid thoughts in class and in other social situations. This remediation augmented the improvements that he had already made in his classroom cognitive functioning, and it also made him more amenable to pursuing social-behavioral interventions. The improvement in his classroom functioning was corroborated by his semester grades, which consolidated his motivation in therapy.

Orientation and Self-Monitoring

Disorientation is a well-known symptom of severe, acute psychiatric disorders, which almost always abates after the acute phase. Occasionally, however, disorientation persists into the residual phase, such as in patients who are poor drug responders, whose clinical presentation is diagnostically anomalous, and/or who have neurological complications. In such cases, chronic disorientation leads to a breakdown in integration of several molecular cognitive functions, including vigilance, selective attention, short-term memory, and executive functions that plan and control simple social behaviors. This breakdown usually precludes meaningful participation in rehabilitation.

It is sometimes useful to identify the cognitive function of self-monitoring as a preliminary treatment target for these patients. Self-monitoring requires the molar integration of a few simple molecular cognitive functions, enough to allow patients to maintain themselves in a minimally meaningful personal and social context. This integration can be accomplished by focusing on the establishment of a short-term memory capacity sufficient for the patients to cue themselves to check their immediate orientation, compare it to a memory of a simple plan for daily activity, and reorient themselves accordingly.

> An example of a treatment program for disorientation comes from the Lincoln Regional Center, where a forty-six-year-old woman with a rapid cycling bipolar disorder, agitation, and pressured and rambling speech was in a behavior modification program that engaged her in basic orientation conversations several times a day. She was asked such questions as What is your name? What did you eat for breakfast? and What is your schedule today? and was reinforced with ward privileges and praise for correct and coherent responses. A time-out from the reinforcement program was successful in reducing her agitation and abusive behavior. Her family was trained to augment the staff's efforts through using similar behavioral contingencies. Within months, her orientation improved to the point where she could resume rehabilitative activities, which her disorientation had precluded for two years.

Concept Formation and Processing

The formation and use of concepts has long been known to be deficient in various psychiatric populations. Recently, interest has focused on schizophrenia and the frontal lobes of the brain, where most cognitive processes are thought to occur. Weinberger, Berman, and Zec (1986) have gone so far as to hypothesize that schizophrenia represents an organic dementia that permanently disables frontal lobe functioning. This hypothesis is controversial for several reasons. It is difficult to localize conceptual functioning in any one region of the brain. Moreover, conceptual impairments are not unique to schizophrenia, and many schizophrenics do not have conceptual impairments. Finally, studies have demonstrated that the performance of schizophrenics on a conceptual task can be improved by training procedures (Spaulding, Storms, Goodrich, and Sullivan, 1986; Summerfeld and others, 1989; Green, Ganzella, Statz, and Vaclav, 1990; Bellack and others, 1990).

The following case study illustrates direct treatment of a conceptual processing deficit:

The patient was a thirty-eight-year-old man, who suffered an initial psychotic episode during military service. In subsequent inpatient and outpatient care in the Veterans Affairs system, an unequivocal clinical picture of paranoid schizophrenia emerged. At one point, in the midst of a delusional psychotic episode, he killed one person. Declared not guilty by reason of insanity, he was committed to the state hospital.

After several years in the hospital security unit without assaultive behavior, he was transferred to the rehabilitation unit. Although his personal and social functioning was generally good, he had considerable difficulty in most of the rehabilitation modalities. In symptom management group, a modality designed to develop comprehensive understanding of one's psychiatric disorder, its symptoms, and environmental stressors, he was particularly incapacitated. After two years, his insight was limited to knowing his diagnosis. He continued to use concrete, largely persecutory explanations of most everything that happened to him. In social interactions he was typically either openly hostile or ingratiating and obsequious. He had a volatile temper and became agitated with the most minor annoyances and frustrations. As part of his vocational rehabilitation plan, he had enrolled in a hotel management correspondence course but had great difficulty with it. His rehabilitation progress had thus been stalled for at least two years.

Testing revealed that although his molecular cognitive functions were well within normal limits, he had severe impairments on the WCST and the Halstead Categories Test. A comprehensive plan for addressing concept formation and manipulation and other aspects of conceptual processing was designed and implemented. This program included the social apperception exercises described by Spaulding, Storms, Goodrich, and Sullivan (1986) and a number of exercises borrowed from special education technology that address categorization, sequencing, and other conceptual skills. A set of concrete criteria for progress in the symptom management group was developed, and achievement of these criteria was linked to ward privileges in a contingency management program.

Treatment continued over a three-year period, concomitant with the rest of his rehabilitation regimen. Testing was repeated at six-month intervals. Within a year, his performance on the WCST was within normal limits. During the second year, the symptom management therapist began to report an accelerating rate of improvement in that group. In the course of a drug titration to a lower dose, he began to experience some prodromal psychotic symptoms, and he quickly and appropriately renegotiated his neuroleptic regimen with his psychiatrist. This behavior was seen as a striking change, as he had previously been quite secretive about his symptoms.

After two and one-half years of cognitive training, his Halstead Categories score fell within normal limits. The special education teacher reported accelerating improvement on the conceptual exercises and renewed vigor in the correspondence course. By the third year after concept training had begun, the patient had graduated from the symptom management group and had obtained his diploma in hotel management. He began a very stressful process of petitioning for release from the hospital, and he handled it well. To date, his discharge plan is well articulated, and he can reasonably expect release within one to two years.

Attributional Processes

Attributions are beliefs about one's self, others, and the causes of events. The formulation and use of beliefs involve integration of perceptual, attentional, conceptual, memory, and executive processes, and so attributional processing lies in the molar range of cognition.

Attributional problems in severely disordered psychiatric patients fall into three categories: symptom-linked, affect-linked, and achievement-linked. Symptom-linked attributions are associated with psychiatric symptoms, especially delusions. These symptoms sometimes respond to drug interventions, but generally they are the most drug-refractory of the positive symptoms of schizophrenia. Affect-linked attributions are beliefs that are closely linked to affective states, such as the cluster of beliefs that constitutes the cognitive component of self-esteem. Affect-linked attributions are the primary treatment targets of cognitive behavior therapy for depression. Achievement-linked attributions are beliefs about the value of independence, autonomy, personal and social success, and, in the context of rehabilitation, the value of personal effort and investment in making a better life. The complaint that a patient "is unmotivated for treatment" frequently reflects an achievement-linked attributional problem.

Techniques developed by Beck (1976) for treating affect-linked attribution problems are well known and are discussed in the next chapter. It should be noted, however, that research in this area has focused on relatively high-functioning patients, and that little is known about the potential usefulness of these techniques in the more severely dysfunctional patients who most often need psychiatric rehabilitation. A notable exception is the work of Perris (this volume). It is clear that patients' levels of self-esteem (and, presumably, other aspects of their affective status) benefit indirectly from success in rehabilitation. More direct treatment for patients whose self-esteem and related beliefs compromise the effectiveness of rehabilitation interventions may be helpful.

The value of direct treatment of delusional beliefs has been reported in well-replicated, controlled, within-subject case studies, in which contingencies of reinforcement and instruction of rational speech were the interventions used (Liberman, Teigen, Patterson, and Baker, 1973; Wong, Massel, Mosk, and Liberman, 1986). Development of the social skill of keeping one's bizarre beliefs to oneself may be another treatment strategy.

Beliefs about the origins of symptoms and other aspects of one's psychiatric disorder represent another kind of symptom-linked attribution, and these may be usefully addressed in rehabilitation. A patient who believes, for example, that auditory hallucinations are simply the voice of the devil may be less able to manage them or use them as prodromal danger signs than is a patient who believes that they are symptoms of a drug-responsive neurophysiological condition. Successful psychoeducational approaches to changing such beliefs have been reported by Johnson, Ross, and Mastria (1977) and Spaulding, Storms, Goodrich, and Sullivan (1986), but a comprehensive, systematic method of intervention has not been developed. Skills-training modules in symptom management and medication management developed by the UCLA Clinical Research Center for Schizophrenia and Psychiatric Rehabilitation are designed to develop relevant skills, but no research has been done on their effects on symptom-linked attributions. This is a potentially valuable but largely unexplored area in psychiatric rehabilitation.

As with affect and self-esteem, the traditional rehabilitation approach to promoting motivational and related achievement-linked attributions has focused on providing success experiences. Contingency management provides a motivational prosthesis but does not necessarily produce self-sustaining motivation. As the following case study illustrates, direct induction of achievement-linked attributions can facilitate the effects of both rehabilitation and contingency management:

> The patient was a twenty-nine-year-old institutionalized man with severe obsessive-compulsive disorder of late adolescent onset. His IQ appeared to be in the normal range. He was transferred to a long-term rehabilitation unit without much expectation of improvement. Despite repeated hospitalizations, his functioning had deteriorated since onset. Normal social behavior had become totally eclipsed by compulsive rituals. At one point compulsions had prevented food intake to the point that he began to show signs of malnutrition and had to be tube-fed. Drug trials of

imipramine, amitriptyline, and fluoxetine were ineffective, and clomipramine produced a barely discernible decrease in the intensity of his compulsive rituals. A behavioral response prevention program only produced a behavior that could not be prevented, compulsive expectoration.

After a year on a restrictive contingency management program that reinforced minimal personal functioning with social contact and ward privileges, the patient managed to earn privileges one or two days per week. When he lost his privileges, he became dejected or aggressive, often requiring restraint. He blamed the staff for victimizing him. Eventually, it became apparent that he was able to comply with his program just enough to attend salient events, such as ward social events and, especially, University of Nebraska football games. Biweekly cognitive therapy sessions began to focus on how it was that he was able to accomplish the bare minimum for privileges. At one point, when shown a graph of his day-to-day performance with salient events marked in, the patient was visibly taken aback. He had not believed that his behavior was under any kind of control, much less the control of events that he valued. He interpreted the graph as a demonstration of his progress, and he even asked to show it to his parents.

Over a number of months his rate of earning privileges gradually increased, which was repeatedly interpreted for him as evidence of increasing control over his behavior. His blaming of staff and his aggression stopped completely. His predominant mood changed from agitation or dejection to sanguinity, even in the face of frustration. He began to show interest in learning self-regulation techniques such as self-talk and relaxation. He began to speculate about what life might be like after discharge from the hospital. The most restrictive parts of his contingency program were discontinued with no increase in compulsive rituals and a continued increase in his ability to attend scheduled activities and classes.

To date, he is fully engaged in a standard skills-training regimen. He has set a discharge date for himself and participates in the planning process. He still engages in a remarkable amount of compulsive ritual, but does so mostly in private, and it does not interfere with his daily schedule.

Social Cognition and Role Performance

At the most molar end of the cognitive range are processes that mediate complex social functioning. This mediation involves integration of many molecular processes of perception, attention, concept formation and manipulation, and response planning and execution. Brenner, Hodel, Kube, and Roder (1987) have developed a group format skills-training modality designed to strengthen many of the molecular components and to facilitate their integration. It is designed to precede conventional social skills training. The modality consists of a number of specific exercises, many of them similar to exercises described in this chapter. The exercises are interwoven with structured group activities to promote their integration into the molar fabric of social cognition. The modality is currently in widespread use in Europe, where early empirical studies have indicated that it facilitates progress in social skills training.

Social role performance is the sustained, integrated use of a set of cognitive and interpersonal skills made meaningful by a social context. The importance of an ability to perform social roles spurred the development of social skills training (Liberman, King, DeRisi, and McCann, 1975; Hogarty, Goldberg, Schooler, and Ulrich, 1974). The integration of skills into a social role requires a molar cognitive representation of the role. Psychiatric rehabilitation usually focuses on development of the specific skills and of the molecular cognitive processes that support the skills. However, more recent techniques of social skills training have emphasized the involvement of the patient in setting long-term and overall rehabilitation goals that are consonant with desired and adaptive social roles (Liberman, DeRisi, and Mueser, 1989). By connecting the arduous and stepwise training of discrete social skills to desired social roles such as "worker," "family member," and "friend," rehabilitation practitioners can enhance patients' motivation and commitment to the skills training program.

Conclusion

Direct treatment of impairments in cognitive functioning can be a useful and sometimes crucial component of comprehensive psychiatric rehabilitation. Effective use of cognitive techniques requires extensive use of specialized assessment methods, including laboratory procedures, because patients have individually unique constellations of cognitive impairments, many of which can be identified only with specialized assessments. Also, *repeated* assessment is necessary to verify the effectiveness of specific interventions.

The case studies described in this chapter illustrate the potential efficacy of utilizing individualized cognitive interventions in conjunction with psychopharmacology, skills training, behavior modification programs, family therapy, and other forms of treatment involved in comprehensive psychiatric rehabilitation. It would be premature to confidently conclude that the improvements in the above case studies are due to the interventions described. Factors such as cumulative medication effects or medication changes, spontaneous remission of symptoms, and even the passage of time may have contributed to patient improvement. Systematic research will eventually provide more information on the relative efficacy of various techniques for various patients, but until then assessment and treatment must proceed through systematic trial and error.

References

Beck, A. T. *Cognitive Therapy and the Emotional Disorders.* New York: International Universities Press, 1976.

Bellack, A., Mueser, K., Morrison, R., Tierny, A., and Podell, K. "Remediation of Cognitive Deficits in Schizophrenia." *American Journal of Psychiatry,* 1990, *147* (12), 1650-1655.

Bowen, L. "Prediction of Schizophrenic Patients' Response to Skill Training with Laboratory Assessment of Attentional Deficits." Unpublished doctoral dissertation, California School of Professional Psychology, Los Angeles, 1988.

Brenner, H. D., Hodel, B., Kube, G., and Roder, V. "Kognitive Therapie bei Schizophrenen: Problemanalyse und Empirische Ergebnisse [Cognitive therapy in schizophrenia: Problem-analysis and empirical study]." *Nervenarzt,* 1987, *58,* 72-83.

Green, M., Ganzella, S., Satz, P., Vaclav, J. "Teaching the Wisconsin Card Sort to Schizophrenic Patients." *Archives of General Psychiatry,* 1990, *47,* 91-92.

Hogarty, G. E., Goldberg, S. C., Schooler, N. R., and Ulrich, R. F. "Drug and Sociotherapy in the Aftercare of Schizophrenic Patients. Part 2: Two-Year Relapse Rates." *Archives of General Psychiatry,* 1974, *31,* 603-608.

Johnson, W., Ross, J., and Mastria, M. "Delusional Behavior: An Attributional Analysis of Development and Modification." *Journal of Abnormal Psychology,* 1977, *86,* 421-426.

Kraemer, S., Zinner, H., and Moller, H. "Cognitive Therapy and Social Skills Training in Chronic Schizophrenia Patients: Preliminary Results of Differential Effects." Paper presented at the 3rd World Congress of Behavior Therapy, Edinburgh, August 1988.

Liberman, R. P., DeRisi, W. J., and Mueser, R. T. *Social Skills Training for Psychiatric Patients.* Elmsford, N.Y.: Pergamon, 1989.

Liberman, R. P., King, L. W., DeRisi, W. J., and McCann, M. J. *Personal Effectiveness.* Champaign, Ill.: Research Press, 1975.

Liberman, R. P., Nuechterlein, K. H., and Wallace, C. J. "Social Skills Training and the Nature of Schizophrenia." In J. Curran and P. Monti (eds.), *Social Skills Training: A Practical Handbook for Assessment and Treatment.* New York: Guilford, 1982.

Liberman, R. P., Teigen, J., Patterson, R., and Baker, V. "Reducing Delusional Speech in Chronic, Paranoid Schizophrenics." *Journal of Applied Behavior Analysis,* 1973, *4,* 273-274.

Nuechterlein, K. H. "Information-Processing Anomalies in the Early Phase of Schizophrenia and Bipolar Disorders." Paper presented at the 4th Annual Society for Research in Psychopathology Conference, Boulder, Colorado, November 1990.

Nuechterlein, K. H., and Dawson, M. E. "Information Processing and Attentional Functioning in the Developmental Course of Schizophrenic Disorders." *Schizophrenia Bulletin,* 1984, *10,* 160-203.

Pogue-Geile, M. F., and Oltmanns, T. F. "Sentence Perception and Distractibility in Schizophrenic, Manic, and Depressed Patients." *Journal of Abnormal Psychology,* 1980, *89,* 115-124.

Spaulding, W. "Spontaneous and Induced Cognitive Changes During Rehabilitation of Schizophrenia." In R. Cromwell (ed.), *Schizophrenia: Innovations in Theory and Treatment.* New York: Oxford University Press, in press.

Spaulding, W., Penn, D., and Weiler, M. "Relationships Between Cognitive and Social Functioning in Chronic Schizophrenia." Paper presented at the 24th Annual American Psychological Association Conference, New York, March 1990.

Spaulding, W., Storms, L., Goodrich, V., and Sullivan, M. "Applications of Experimental Psychopathology in Psychiatric Rehabilitation." *Schizophrenia Bulletin,* 1986, *12,* 560-577.

Spivak, G., Platt, S., and Shure, M. *The Problem-Solving Approach to Adjustment.* San Francisco: Jossey-Bass, 1976.

Spohn, H., and Strauss, M. "Relation of Neuroleptic and Anticholinergic Medication to Cognitive Functions in Schizophrenia." *Journal of Abnormal Psychology,* 1989, *98,* 367-380.

Summerfeld, A., Alphs, L., Wagman, A., Funderburk, F., and Strauss, M. "Monetary Reinforcement Reduces Perseverative Errors in Patients with Schizophrenia." Paper presented at the 2nd International Congress on Schizophrenia Research, San Diego, California, April 1989.

Weinberger, D. R., Berman, K. F., and Zec, R. F. "Physiological Dysfunction of Dorsolateral Prefrontal Cortex in Schizophrenia. Part 1: Regional Cerebral Blood Flow Evidence." *Archives of General Psychiatry*, 1986, *43*, 114–124.

Wong, S. E., Massel, H. K., Mosk, M. D., and Liberman, R. P. "Behavioral Approaches to the Treatment of Schizophrenia." In G. D. Burrows, T. R. Norman, and G. Rubinstein (eds.), *Handbook of Studies of Schizophrenia*. Amsterdam, Holland: Elsevier, 1986.

DORIE REED, Ph.D., is a clinical psychologist and research associate in the Department of Psychology at the University of Nebraska at Lincoln. She provides cognitive therapy on the extended care rehabilitation unit at the Lincoln Regional Center where the research reported in this chapter was done.

MARY E. SULLIVAN, M.S.W., is director of the extended care rehabilitation unit at the Lincoln Regional Center where she also conducts therapy and supervises social work services.

DAVID L. PENN is a graduate student in the Department of Psychology at the University of Nebraska at Lincoln.

PAUL STUVE, Ph.D., was a graduate student at the Department of Psychology at the University of Nebraska and is now program director at the Rehabilitation Unit of Broughton State Hospital in North Carolina.

WILLIAM D. SPAULDING, Ph.D., is associate professor of psychology at the University of Nebraska at Lincoln and chief psychologist at the extended care rehabilitation unit at the Lincoln Regional Center.

The multidetermined nature of the disability of patients suffering from schizophrenic disorders requires a comprehensive treatment approach that includes cognitive-behavioral therapy.

A Cognitive-Behavioral Treatment Program for Patients with a Schizophrenic Disorder

Carlo Perris

A comprehensive and individualized cognitive-behavioral treatment program, developed for young persons suffering from schizophrenic disorders, has been developed at the University of Umea in Northern Sweden (Perris, 1989a). The program is located in ordinary houses in the community, where six patients per home live in a family-like atmosphere, providing for themselves in daily chores, shopping, and preparation of meals.

The staff at each center comprises seven full-time mental health nurses working on a day-time schedule, one full-time occupational therapist, and one part-time physiotherapist. All personnel were intensively trained in cognitive psychotherapy (Perris, 1989b). One mental health nurse at each center rotates the night duty, while I, as the senior doctor, have the medical responsibility of all three centers. I act also as the director of the treatment program in general, and supervise the individual therapy sessions one afternoon a week at each center. Two therapists, chosen at each center from among the nurses who are responsible for the individual therapy sessions, are assigned to each patient. To facilitate the integration of the various treatment components, both the occupational therapist and the physiotherapist regularly participate in the supervision sessions.

Patients and Their Recruitment. Priority is given to patients in the age range of eighteen to thirty-five years who meet a DSM-III-R diagnosis of schizophrenic disorder, independently of whether they are still presenting psychotic symptoms or are in remission. Patients suffering from an Axis II personality disorder are, occasionally, also accepted into the

NEW DIRECTIONS FOR MENTAL HEALTH SERVICES, no. 53, Spring 1992 © Jossey-Bass Publishers program. Excluded are patients with verified brain damage who are judged unable to participate in a verbal therapy program. Patients with a history of prolonged alcohol or substance dependence and patients with a history of documented and repeated violence are also excluded. Since participation in the treatment program is voluntary, the patient must be prepared to stay at a center for the period of treatment that is stipulated in the initial contract and to accept the general conditions of the program.

Patients referred for treatment are discussed at a case conference at the center that expects to have a vacancy in the near future. When a decision has been reached on the possible acceptance of a certain patient, two of the nurse therapists make initial contact and invite the patient to visit the center to form his or her own judgment about the proposed treatment. Patients who appear to be ambivalent might spend a few days at the center as a trial before making their final decisions. For practical reasons, the treatment program has been divided into periods or terms of approximately six months. While the aim is to obtain a fair distribution of patients according to sex and most prominent symptomatology, neither of those distributional criteria can always be strictly met.

Problem Inventory and the Treatment Contract. Within the very first days at a center, an inventory of the patient's problems is conducted with the focus of the assessment on areas of functioning and on what the patient expects to achieve, rather than on symptoms. Also, a preliminary assessment is made of which solutions to his or her problems the patient has adopted in the past, and of the reasons for their possible failure. Symptoms are, whenever possible, reformulated in terms of problems to be solved, at the same time as a first attempt is made to make the patient aware of a possible relationship between his or her symptomatology and problems in other areas of social functioning.

The following excerpt from an assessment interview illustrates the problem-focused nature of the evaluation:

THERAPIST: What is your major problem right now?
PATIENT: I don't have any place to live in. I must get a flat or something.
THERAPIST: Have you ever lived on your own?
PATIENT: Oh yes! I have rented a flat on several occasions.
THERAPIST: Why is it that you don't have any right now?
PATIENT: Well . . . It was every time the same problem. . . . The other tenants in the houses where I lived were hostile.
THERAPIST: How did they manifest their hostility?
PATIENT: They made noises to disturb me. . . . You know . . . I'm sure that they were spying on me.
THERAPIST: Has it been a similar pattern in all the places where you have lived?
PATIENT: It's become worse during the last few years. . . . I've had to change apartments at least three times.

THERAPIST: Did you have any difficulty in changing apartments?

PATIENT: Well . . . no. . . . People at the social welfare have fixed it for me.

THERAPIST: Would you be able to get a new apartment by yourself?

PATIENT: I don't know . . . I never tried.

THERAPIST: Well, let me summarize. It seems to me that you have voiced three different problems. The first is that you need a new flat to live in. Second, you experience hostility from the other tenants at the places where you live. And, third, you would have some difficulty in trying by yourself to rent a new flat. Right?

PATIENT: It seems so.

THERAPIST: Would it help you if we worked together on all three of those problems?

PATIENT: I don't know. . . . What I need is a new flat where nobody will disturb me.

THERAPIST: Okay. We will give the issue of getting a flat a top priority. On the other hand, how would you feel if this time everything went well and you did not get into any further trouble with your neighbors?

PATIENT: I would feel great.

THERAPIST: Do you think that it would help you if we looked together at what happened on the previous occasions?

PATIENT: If you say so.

THERAPIST: It would be nice if we could look a little closer at your opinions about the behavior of your neighbors to see if there is any solution suitable for you. Also, you could devote part of your time while here at the center in training to how to rent a flat when in need. That would make you even more independent in the future.

In this case example, the therapist collects information both on the presented problem (that is, lack of a flat) and on the reasons why the patient is presently homeless (that is, a paranoid attitude toward the neighbors). Also, the therapist can recognize the patient's lack of appropriate skills for renting a flat. However, by agreeing on the goal expressed by the patient, the therapist engages in a first attempt to make the patient aware of other problems that also need appropriate solutions. Note that, at this stage, no attempt is made to challenge the patient's delusional beliefs.

At the end of the inventory, and when an agreement has been reached on some preliminary goal, the patient is asked to sign a contract for at least one six-month term. The contract stipulates the main rules concerning the patient's stay at the center, for example, the duties to keep one's own room in order and to participate in the various treatment activities and details about time that can be spent out of the center. Also in the contract is a formal consent to participate in video-recorded therapy sessions and in the ongoing evaluation program.

Even though the initial contract does not cover a period longer than one term, the majority of patients remain for additional periods. According to a patient's motivation, and when a fair possibility of achieving more important goals is envisaged, the treatment contract is renewed for one term at a time. On average, most of the patients remain at the centers for about three terms or one and one-half years. Whenever necessary, follow-ups of various lengths on an outpatient basis are also planned. In each case, the therapists who have been in charge of a patient at a particular center are responsible also for the continuation of therapy during the follow-up. Even when a patient does not need any further immediate contact after discharge, booster meetings are planned at six months, at one year, and at two years after discharge.

Goals of Treatment and Concurrent Medication. While the major goals of the treatment centers are improving functional self-representations, mastering social skills, and producing a more realistic perspective of the future, concurrent psychotropic medications are administered routinely. Because of the successful engagement of patients in cognitive-behavioral treatment, it has been possible to progressively reduce the dosages of antipsychotic medication to low levels. Patients work collaboratively with the psychiatrist and their therapists to experiment with drug dosages in order to become convinced of their usefulness; thus, patients' adherence to their drug regimes comes through their own convictions rather than by imposition. Moreover, patients learn to become attentive to changes in their stress levels, symptoms, and side effects that direct them to negotiate changes in their drug treatment.

Components of the Treatment Program

A multilevel treatment program is implemented at each center, including (1) a *milieu therapeutic level,* with training in daily life skills and interpersonal relations, (2) a *group level* comprising weekly sessions, (3) a consistent use of *nonverbal therapeutic strategies* by the occupational therapist and the physiotherapist, both in groups and individually, and (4) an *individual level* comprising weekly individual psychotherapy sessions. In addition, patients are encouraged, in the form of "homework" assignments, to become involved in various activities in the community during their stay at the center. Finally, *psychosocial interventions with family members* are also planned, both on an informal basis and as a part of a special research program.

Milieu Therapeutic Level of Intervention. Life at the centers is organized in a family life fashion, enhanced by the presence of pet animals whose therapeutic relevance has been repeatedly emphasized in the literature (Beck and Katcher, 1984; Perris, 1989a). The guiding principles of the daily program derive from milieu therapy, Bowlby's (1979, 1988) concept of a secure base, and the major tenets of cognitive therapy. Bowlby has emphasized that human beings of all ages are able to use their talents to

best advantage when they are confident that standing behind
trusted persons who will come to their aid should difficulties ari
trusted persons at the centers are the patients' therapists, who pr
patients with a secure base from which to operate.

The more general "cognitive therapy attitude" that permeates the whole
atmosphere at the centers and rules the interaction of staff and patients
has been described in detail elsewhere (Perris, 1989a, b). Primarily, it consists of the development of what Beck (1976) has defined as a relationship
based on "collaborative empiricism." To develop this kind of relationship,
therapists and patients are expected to actively work together, as if they
were two research workers, in the definition of problems and in the search
of appropriate solutions by putting forward hypotheses and testing their
tenability. In addition to collaborative empiricism, other important principles that characterize our cognitive therapy attitude are summarized in
Exhibit 2.1. In practice, the milieu therapeutic approach takes advantage
of the daily interactions between therapists and patients and those that
occur among the patients themselves. At the same time, the patients' participation in all of the daily chores at the centers constitutes direct training
in ordinary social and family style life.

One major difference between a simple behavioral training program
and the training program at our centers is that the former is primarily
based on the training of new, presumably more adaptive, behaviors,
whereas our cognitive approach focuses on the identification and correc-
tion of dysfunctional cognitions that previously hampered the development
and use of appropriate abilities. During everyday life at the centers, cognitive restructuring occurs in spontaneous staff-patient interactions; furthermore, therapists' observations of the behavior of patients can be easily
integrated into the more formal group and individual cognitive therapy
sessions, as described below.

Exhibit 2.1. Principles Implicit in Cognitive Therapy and the Attitudes of Cognitive Therapists

Developing a collaborative empiricism

Accepting the basic tenets of cognitive therapy concerning the relationship among
thoughts, emotions, and behavior and their reciprocal influence

Taking into account the singularity of each patient, independently of present status or
diagnostic categorization

Addressing the healthy aspects of the patient rather than focusing on symptoms

Trusting that every individual has a potential of being able to influence his or her own
condition, at least to a certain extent

Promoting the development and maintenance of the patient's autonomy

Promoting the unfolding and enhancement of the patient's competence

Group Activities. Group activities are scheduled weekly and comprise special sessions with the physiotherapist and the occupational therapist as well as formal group therapy sessions. Group activities with the physiotherapist are mostly of a recreational and sports nature, while activities led by the occupational therapist comprise art therapy and the planning and preparation of meals, shopping, and budgets. Creative painting can provide a first glimpse into patients who have difficulty expressing themselves verbally.

The more formal group therapy sessions occur twice weekly. One session is devoted to the training of social skills. In this context we take into account the three aspects of interpersonal problem-solving skills conceptualized by Liberman and others (1986): *receiving, processing,* and *sending skills.* Access to naturalistic observations of the patients' behavior both at the centers and in the community, and the results of both staff and self-ratings obtained at admission, permit staff to pinpoint the skills that each patient needs to learn. Also, a special manual covering ten sessions has been developed as a semistandardized set of guidelines for social skills training. There is one major difference between a more behavioristic approach to social skills training and our approach based on cognitive therapy principles. The more behavioristic approach, as exemplified by Liberman, DeRisi, and Mueser (1989), teaches skills through behavioral rehearsal or repetition of a statement until the patient makes an appropriate response, which is then rewarded and reinforced. From a cognitive therapy viewpoint, the focus is primarily on questioning the patient about what inhibits him or her in giving an appropriate response and on challenging dysfunctional cognitions related to such inhibition; subsequent to these cognitive interventions, the patient is encouraged to give the response that he or she feels is appropriate and is coached on its appropriateness. Also, instead of an external reward, we try, as far as possible, to help the patient find within himself or herself the primary source of reward.

The following hypothetical, highly condensed excerpt, constructed to match the example reported by Liberman, DeRisi, and Mueser (1989, p. 194), illustrates the training procedure:

LARS: I bought this shirt yesterday.
EVA: [no response]
THERAPIST: Eva, did you notice Lars's new shirt?
EVA: Yes.
THERAPIST: Do you like it?
EVA: Yes.
THERAPIST: Would you like to tell Lars that you approve of his new shirt?
EVA: I don't know.
THERAPIST: How do you think Lars would react if you told him that his new shirt is nice?
EVA: [no response]

THERAPIST: Is anything going on in your mind?

EVA: I think that I would be intrusive if I commented on Lars's shirt.

THERAPIST: If you had bought a new shirt and Lars were telling you that it was nice, would you feel intruded upon?

EVA: I don't think so.

THERAPIST: Is there any reason why Lars should be different and feel that you were intruding on him?

EVA: No . . . I don't know.

THERAPIST: Would it be too much for you to make a try?

EVA: [With a somewhat slurred speech] Lars, your new shirt is very nice.

LARS: That was kind of you Eva.

THERAPIST: How do you feel having been able to say what you wanted?

EVA: Good.

THERAPIST: How would you have felt if you had not said what you wanted to say?

EVA: I would have felt to be a failure as in so many previous occasions.

THERAPIST: Well, if it makes you feel good to say what you would like to say, what could you do now?

EVA: Say it again. [Turning to Lars and with a clearer voice] You have bought a shirt that suits you very well, Lars.

It must be emphasized, however, that the excerpt reported by Liberman, DeRisi, and Mueser concerned a patient with a schizophrenic disorder who had been hospitalized for several years and was socially isolated for a long time. With patients of that type, it might be appropriate to start social skills training at a more elementary, behavioral level. However, a shift to a more cognitive-behavioral sequence of training should be made whenever collaborative participation of the patients can be foreseen. Preliminary, unpublished results concerning our approach suggest that the special skills taught in the group sessions do generalize to situations outside the centers; also, the acquired skills appear to be maintained for at least one year after the end of the treatment program. During the training sessions described above, appropriate behavioral techniques such as role play, rehearsal, modeling, and social reinforcement are consistently used.

The other formal group session, though closely related to social skills training, is specifically focused on the identification, differentiation, and expression of feelings and emotions. One recurring theme in this group concerns the distinction among irritation, anger, and aggression and their identification and appropriate expression. Other themes discussed in this group are the differentiation among feeling down, feeling sad, or being depressed, and between occasional feelings of tension and the experience of anxiety. Patients are encouraged to pinpoint situations in which they would have liked to express (or have expressed) some feeling, and a discussion follows on the appropriateness of the emotion and of its expression.

Also, the therapists can suggest the pinpointing of situations that have occurred at the center as a starting point for discussion. In this particular type of group session, pictures from magazines or slides are used to train the patients in recognizing emotional states. Also, appropriate bibliotherapy is accessible for selected readings. As in other center activities, the general conduct of the session is based on cognitive therapy principles and on techniques such as role play, modeling, and guided imagery.

A group session is held every Friday to summarize the past week and coach the patients on making plans for the weekend. Both positive and negative experiences are elicited in order to reinforce the former and mitigate the impact of the latter. In planning weekend events, patients are encouraged to choose activities outside of the center. Guided imagery is used to prepare them for possible success, or failure, in their planning.

Individual Therapy Sessions. Individual sessions are scheduled with a frequency that varies according to the needs of each patient and to the phase of treatment. However, two weekly sessions is the general rule. Great flexibility by the therapist is required both in the planning and in the conduct of the sessions. Such flexibility concerns both the frequency and the length of the sessions, and their pace. Other general rules require the therapist to address the healthy aspects of the patient's personality in order to discourage regressive reactions, and to move sequentially from topics that are peripheral toward those that are more emotionally laden.

We prefer to begin with problems that the patient experiences in the "here and now," and that can be managed with a certain probability of success, taking into account the patient's present resources. Solutions to problems that at first glance may appear of negligible importance in the whole pattern of the patient's total disability represent most often a first step toward enhancement of the patient's self-esteem and reinforce both his or her motivation for treatment and the therapeutic relationship. The main focus of the therapeutic sessions, however, is on the task of challenging the cognitive distortions presented by the patient. Distortions that occur frequently are desymbolization, lack of awareness of asymmetry in human relations, egocentric overinclusiveness, and predicate thinking.

Hallucinatory and delusional experiences are addressed with the basic principles of cognitive therapy (for details, see Perris, 1989a). First, the patient is made aware that he or she is able to exert at least some control over such experiences. Second, efforts are directed at modifying the interference and pervasiveness of the pathological experiences, and the preoccupation that they cause. Finally, the patient is guided toward recognition that those very experiences are intimately related to his or her own thoughts, fantasies, and expectations.

The following excerpt of an interview illustrates how a female patient at an early stage of treatment was trained to exert some control over hallucinatory experiences thought to be completely beyond her control.

EVA: [tense and anxious] Please, help me. . . . I am continuously disturbed by frightening, accusing voices. . . . I cannot control them. . . . I'm going to be completely crazy.

THERAPIST: Do you hear those voices now, when you speak to me?

EVA: No . . . not now . . . but at all other times.

THERAPIST: Is there any occasion when you are less disturbed by those voices?

EVA: Well . . . occasionally when I'm in the living room together with the other patients.

THERAPIST: And when are they at their worst?

EVA: When I'm alone in my room. . . . They're terrible.

THERAPIST: It seems to me that you are most disturbed when you are alone and a little less disturbed when you are in the living room together with the other patients. Is that correct?

EVA: Yes.

THERAPIST: Well . . . tell me, who decides whether you stay in your room, or you go to the living room?

EVA: [surprised] Why do you ask? . . . It's me who decides.

THERAPIST: Do you remember that you have said that you were less disturbed by "the voices" when you were in the living room?

EVA: Yes . . . only for a short time.

THERAPIST: Okay. Even though it might be for only a short time, what could you do to be less disturbed by the voices?

EVA: Be in the living room.

THERAPIST: Correct. And who decides your being in the living room?

EVA: It's me.

THERAPIST: Then it seems to me that you can decide to be in the living room and accordingly to be less disturbed by the voices. Is that so?

EVA: Yes.

THERAPIST: Would you agree that if things are as we have just discussed, you can exert some control over the voices?

EVA: Well . . . maybe. . . . I don't know. . . . You are probably right.

In the course of the therapeutic sessions, consistent use is made of the techniques and strategies of cognitive psychotherapy (see Perris, 1989a, for a thorough description of these strategies and techniques). Some of the main components of the therapeutic process are summarized in Figure 2.1.

Homework. Homework assignments are consistently used throughout the whole treatment program. Homework can concern tasks to be carried out at a center (for example, suggested readings and completion of the forms and self-ratings that are a part of the ongoing evaluation program) or tasks of various complexity to be carried out in the community (for example, making and keeping appointments with social agencies, getting in touch with people). The results of homework assignments are consistently reviewed in the next individual session, following the routine principles of

Figure 2.1. Main Components of the Therapeutic Processes Leading to Cognitive Restructuring

Distancing

Reattribution

Development of metacognition

Decentering

Neutralization of negative automatic thoughts

Challenging of cognitive distortions

Training of interpersonal skills

Modification of basic meaning structures

cognitive therapy. Toward the end of treatment, for example, when a patient is preparing to move into his or her own flat, homework assignments may concern the furnishing of the flat, and planning evenings and having guests.

Contacts with Patients' Relatives. Relatives of the patients are encouraged to visit the centers. On those occasions, informal meetings occur with the patients' therapists. Since we make a consistent distinction between *attachment* and *dependence,* we counteract the latter but respect the former. Hence, patients are encouraged to become independent but also to remain attached to their parents. At the family meetings, efforts are made to promote a more functional interaction between the patient and his or her visiting relatives, at the same time as confrontation is discouraged. With select relatives a controlled research program has been implemented that takes into account an assessment of "expressed emotion" (Imber-Mintz and others, 1987) and comprises six standard psychoeducational sessions.

Ongoing Evaluation. At admission, and later at scheduled intervals, the patients participate in planned evaluations. This program comprises the collection of selected video-recorded sessions at the beginning and end of each term and the completion of a battery of rating instruments. Those instruments are both ratings made by the staff and self-ratings completed by the patients. They include ratings of psychopathology, ratings of various cognitive variables (for example, dysfunctional assumptions, automatic negative thoughts, cognitive distortions, deployment of attention), and ratings of social functioning and interpersonal contacts. So far, only a few preliminary evaluative data have been reported (Perris, Toresson, and others, 1990; Perris, Nordstrom, and Troeng, in press). We have refrained from reporting more extensive evaluation results because we wish to have at least two-year follow-up data to assess the durability of our clinical results. Also, we expect that the development of similar centers in other parts of Sweden will allow for a more rapid collection of outcome data with a larger series of patients. In general, it can be stated that less than 5 percent of patients either do not profit from the treatment program or drop out of treatment. The majority appear to be able to achieve improved cognitive functioning and a satisfactorily high level of social functioning; for example, 90 percent have been able to move into their own apartments, and 60 percent are currently at work or in school.

Conclusion

The comprehensive cognitive-behavioral treatment program in small, family style residences is particularly suitable for young patients suffering from schizophrenic disorders who are not yet "burned-out." In our clinical experience since 1986, the intensive and individualized rehabilitation effort permits the achievement of satisfactory, long-lasting results with a sizable proportion of these carefully selected, young, verbally competent, and cooperative patients.

The program can be applied at small community-based treatment units, psychiatric hospitals that permit partial hospitalization, and day centers. The utilization of nurse therapists in the key clinical roles appears to contain the costs of treatment within reasonable limits. One prerequisite of program implementation is competent, intensive supervision based on principles and procedures of cognitive therapy.

References

Beck, A. T. *Cognitive Therapy and the Emotional Disorders.* New York: International Universities Press, 1976.

Beck, A. T., and Katcher, A. H. "A New Look at Pet-Facilitated Therapy." *Journal of the American Veterinary Medicine Association,* 1984, *184,* 414–421.

Bowlby, J. "Self-Reliance and Some Conditions That Promote It." In J. Bowlby (ed.), *The Making and Breaking of Affectional Bonds.* London, England: Tavistock, 1979.

Bowlby, J. *A Secure Base: Parent-Child Attachment and Healthy Human Development.* Basic Books, 1988.

Imber-Mintz, L., Liberman, R. P., Miklowitz, D. J., and Mintz, J. "Expressed Emotion: A Clarion Call for Research and a Partnership for Education Among Practitioners, Patients, Families, and Administrators." *Schizophrenia Bulletin,* 1987, *13,* 227–235.

Liberman, R. P., DeRisi, W. J., and Mueser, K. T. *Social Skills Training for Psychiatric Patients.* Elmsford, N.Y.: Pergamon, 1989.

Liberman, R. P., Mueser, K. T., Wallace, C. J., Jacobs, H. E., Eckman, T. A., and Massel, H. K. "Training Skills in the Psychiatrically Disabled: Learning, Coping, and Competence." *Schizophrenia Bulletin,* 1986, *12,* 631–647.

Perris, C. *Cognitive Therapy with Schizophrenic Patients.* New York: Guilford, 1989a.

Perris, C. Personalinriktad utbilning i kognitiv psykoterapi med sarskild hansyn till utbildningen av personal vid sma psykoterapeutiska enheter for patienter med psykotiska syndrome [Cognitive psychotherapy personalized in a psychotherapeutic center for patients with psychosis]. Reports of the Department of Psychiatry, New Series, no. 1. Umea, Sweden: Umea University, 1989b.

Perris, C., Nordstrom, G., and Troeng, L. "A Three-Year Cognitive-Behavioral Treatment of a Young Woman Suffering from a Schizophrenic Disorder." In A. Freeman and F. M. Dattilio (eds.), Casebook in Cognitive-Behavior Therapy. New York: Plenum, in press.

Perris, C., Toresson, P., Skagerlind, L., Warburton, E., Gustavsson, H., and Johansson, T. "Integrating Components in a Comprehensive Cognitive Treatment Program for Patients with a Schizophrenic Disorder." In C. N. Stefanis and others (eds.), Psychiatry: A World Perspective. Amsterdam, Holland: Elsevier, 1990.

CARLO PERRIS, M.D., is professor of psychiatry and chair of the Department of Psychiatry, University of Umea, and director of the WHO Collaborating Center for Research and Training in Mental Health, Umea, Sweden. He is president of the Swedish Society of Cognitive Psychotherapy and Research.

A clinical research program for persons suffering from schizophrenia has been designed to optimize the additive effects of social skills training and assertive case management.

Combining Social Skills Training and Assertive Case Management: The Social and Independent Living Skills Program of the Brentwood Veterans Affairs Medical Center

Jerome V. Vaccaro, Robert P. Liberman, Charles J. Wallace, Gayla Blackwell

Changes in the focus and locus of care for persons with serious mental disorders have spurred the development of two new modes of treatment and rehabilitation: case management and social skills training. Case management became important as individuals with chronic mental illness were deinstitutionalized from the large state hospitals in which they previously resided. Some of the first truly comprehensive efforts in this regard were reported by Stein and Test (1980) in their descriptions of the Training in Community Living and Program of Assertive Community Treatment model. In this approach, teams of clinicians take responsibility for the compre-

The project on which this chapter is based is supported in part by a research grant from the VA Health Services Research and Development Service awarded to R. P. Liberman, M.D. (principal investigator) at the Rehabilitation Medicine Service of the Brentwood (Psychiatric) Division of the West Los Angeles VA Medical Center. We acknowledge the following individuals, whose hard work and dedication made this project successful: Berniece Allen, Ronald Allen, George Bartzokis, Mitchell Caine, Martin Cohen, Mark Eisner, Ethel Kleinschmidt, Sumie Kumagai, Sondra Levine, Edgar Mitchell, Kathryn Moe, Ann Powell, Carol Reimer, Greer Sullivan, Andre Trinh, and Sonia Vellani.

hensive community care of chronically mentally ill individuals. They assertively advocate these individuals' needs, helping them successfully make the transition from lives wholly dependent on others to lives in which they assume greater responsibility for and autonomy in their self-care. In these programs, clinicians deliver services in the streets, shops, and residences of the community, seeking out their patients rather than waiting for them to appear in clinics or hospitals. Researchers have now demonstrated the replicability of this model (Allness, Knoedler, and Test, 1985; Test, 1991), and Witheridge (1989) has addressed the training needs for staff who engage in these efforts.

Case Management and Social Skills Training

Over the past decade, social skills training has gained widespread acceptance as an effective psychosocial treatment in the care of individuals with chronic mental illness (Liberman, Mueser, and Wallace, 1986; Benton and Schroeder, 1990). This method involves the systematic application of behavioral learning techniques targeted to help individuals gain the knowledge and skills that they need to perform in social settings. Skills necessary for such competencies as establishing and maintaining friendships, dating, holding conversations, self-managing medications and symptoms, and grooming and self-care have been successfully taught (Liberman, 1988). Typically, these interventions are delivered in group settings according to prescribed practices and in some cases are organized into formal curricula or modules (Wallace, Boone, Donahoe, and Foy, 1985).

The Social and Independent Living Skills Program

Clinical services in this program are comprehensive in scope because patients require a broad array of services, including psychopharmacological management, psychosocial therapies such as social skills training, and various measures to meet basic needs. These services are woven together into a continuous fabric through the use of case management in the Social and Independent Living Skills program. The 110 patients in the program are served by a multidisciplinary staff led by senior clinicians who are experts in working with the seriously mentally disabled.

Goal-Setting and Treatment and Rehabilitation Planning. Efforts to treat and rehabilitate individuals with chronic mental illnesses are doomed to failure unless they are linked to self-identified goals and desired life roles (Vaccaro, Pitts, and Wallace, 1991). All too often, we plan our interventions without even soliciting the input of our patients. While our current effort falls somewhat short in this regard, it is important to highlight the process by which we obtain information about impairment, disability, and handicap for purposes of treatment planning.

It is useful to separate the evaluation process into two overlapping but distinct procedures: diagnostic and functional assessments. In the former, one gathers data in the service of generating a diagnostic formulation. These data usually include information about symptoms, social functioning, and family history. It is particularly important to identify the symptoms and rate them in severity so that they can be monitored and used to guide long-term clinical decision making, especially in regard to medication (Lukoff, Ventura, Liberman, and Nuechterlein, 1991). However, in many treatment settings, little or no attention is paid to the issues related to the goals or important life roles that patients identify for themselves, the skills that they possess that facilitate their achievement of these ambitions, and the behavioral deficits or disturbances that impede this growth. These data, collectively seen as the material of a functional assessment, guide treatment and rehabilitative efforts in the Social and Independent Living Skills program. They are of particular value in social skills training and rehabilitation-focused case management (Kuehnel and Liberman, 1988).

In our program, patients, upon entry, are assigned a case manager and a psychiatrist, who then oversee the completion of these assessments. The assessments are seen as "works in progress" and are continually updated. Functional assessment data are obtained through the use of the Independent Living Skills Survey (Wallace, 1986) and through direct observation and are summarized in each patient's "Individualized Written Rehabilitation Plan." An important component of this process of data collection and summarization is the identification by the patients of incentives that they feel would reinforce their participation in treatment and rehabilitation. These incentives might include travel money, articles of clothing, food, and books. These items are then employed as "reinforcers" that spur continued involvement.

Case Management. All patients receive clinical case management, which can be characterized as assertive and intensive. Many activities are performed in the community, with case managers assisting patients in the tasks of defining and meeting patients' needs. Case managers thus seek out patients instead of passively waiting for them to appear for services. In addition, the case managers are psychologists or social workers with advanced degrees who are equipped to accurately assess psychopathology and warning signs of relapse and to provide behaviorally oriented services in vivo. Patients in the Social and Independent Living Skills program are encouraged by their case managers to use the structured problem-solving techniques that they learn in skills training classes whenever they have needs or problems. This process is designed to provoke greater generalization of learned skills (Vaccaro and Liberman, 1989).

Psychopharmacological Treatment. Patients are seen on a regular basis by a psychiatrist for medication monitoring. Emphasis is placed on their understanding of the indications for and complications of their medications, and on their recognition that they must be active partners in the process of medication prescription and monitoring (Corrigan, Liberman, and Engel, 1990). Attempts are made to titrate medications to their lowest effective doses, based on the assumptions that more is not necessarily better and that enhanced compliance results from better balances between benefits and side effects of medications (Van Putten and Marder, 1987). Symptom monitoring and medication titration are guided through the use of structured instruments such as the Brief Psychiatric Rating Scale (BPRS) and the Abnormal Involuntary Movement Scale (AIMS).

Social Skills Training. Psychiatric rehabilitation comprises two sets of overlapping activities: helping patients develop or reacquire social and instrumental skills, and developing supportive environments for patients. Social skills training is delivered in our program in group settings, using the Social and Independent Living Skills Modules developed by Liberman and colleagues at the University of California-Los Angeles Clinical Research Center for Schizophrenia and Psychiatric Rehabilitation (available from Psychiatric Rehabilitation Consultants, P. O. Box 6620, Camarillo, Calif. 93011-6620).

All patients receive competency-based instruction in four core skill areas: medication management, symptom management, basic conversation, and recreation and leisure. Classes are run four days per week, three hours per day, for a period of six months. Each of the classes is sixty to seventy-five minutes in length. The total length of instruction varies slightly from group to group, since cohorts do not proceed to the next skill area until the material is learned. Ongoing progress is monitored through the use of "pop quizzes" administered during and after the social skills training classes. Patients are further assessed for knowledge and skills acquisition and maintenance at the end of the six-month intensive treatment phase and every six to twelve months thereafter. Therapists' competency and adherence to the model is regularly assessed as well, ensuring high degrees of fidelity to the model.

Continuous Treatment. It is our firm conviction that sustained clinical efforts are required for treatment and rehabilitation gains to be cumulative and maintained over time. Once our patients complete the first six months of skills training, they enter into the generalization phase of the program. Case management efforts are directed toward helping patients generalize the skills learned in the classroom to other life areas. All patients periodically update their Individualized Written Rehabilitation Plans, the framework for which is shown in Exhibit 3.1. These plans address goals in major life domains such as housing and household maintenance, symptomatic status, occupation, social and family life, and finances.

Case managers use behavioral learning interventions such as structured problem solving and role play in their practice, as illustrated in the following case vignette.

Exhibit 3.1. Excerpt from the Individualized Written Rehabilitation Plan, Delineating Questions Used to Develop Goals in the Vocational Domain

1. What are the patient's desired vocational roles and goals?
2. What is the patient's current vocational functioning?
   a. Status (competitive employment, supported employment, unemployed)
   b. Adequacy: How does the patient's current vocational status *enhance or assist* his or her current functioning? For example, what vocational skills make him or her employable?
   c. Adequacy: How does the patient's current vocational status *impede or interfere with* his or her current functioning? For example, what skills does he or she lack that preclude employment?
3. What are the expected benefits of changing or maintaining the patient's vocational status?
4. What are the patient's personal resources that enhance attainment of these goals?
5. What are the patient's personal obstacles that impede goal attainment?
6. What are the patient's environmental resources that enhance attainment of these goals?
7. What are the patient's environmental obstacles that impede attainment of these goals?
8. Detailed plan to achieve these goals:

Bill is a thirty-four-year-old man, diagnosed as schizophrenic, who entered the Social and Independent Living Skills program after many years of psychiatric treatment that he characterized as unhelpful. He had been hospitalized on average two to three times per year over the preceding six years and had been largely resistant to staying on medication and accepting other forms of treatment. He told his case manager that he wanted to leave the board-and-care home in which he presently resided because it was in an unsafe neighborhood.

Bill's case manager helped him clarify and solve this problem according to a seven-step problem-solving process (Liberman, 1988). Bill had been introduced to this process during his involvement in the skills training modules. Bill decided that he would like to live in a particular board-and-care home, and that he would set up an appointment with its operator to interview for a place in the home. He and his case manager then role played this interview so that he felt comfortable with his performance and ability to assert his own needs. His case manager offered modeling of appropriate assertiveness skills and abundant praise for Bill's role-play effort.

Next, Bill and his case manager agreed that he would call the operator for an appointment. He did so and planned the materials and resources that he would need to be successful in this endeavor. For example, he called the bus company to get their route schedule, made sure he had appropriate change for the fare, and put together an outfit of suitable clothing. When the appointment time came, Bill felt that he was well prepared and confident. He met with the operator and they agreed that he could live in the home for the two weeks before his first disability check was to arrive. Bill has now been living in this board-and-care home for the past six months and continues to use the problem-solving process with reinforcement and coaching from his case manager to deal with problems such as making new friends, enrolling in a vocational rehabilitation program, and reestablishing contact with his family.

Empirical Evaluation

As empirically documented, chronically mentally ill individuals are able to learn and retain new information presented in the skills-training modules used in the Social and Independent Living Skills program (Eckman, Liberman, Phipps, and Blair, 1990). In addition, it has been demonstrated that skills training and similar interventions reduce relapse and recidivism rates (Liberman, Mueser, and Wallace, 1986; Hogarty and others, 1986; Benton and Schroeder, 1990). In the current clinical research effort, we are interested in replicating these findings, and we are also seeking to learn whether such changes affect other variables such as overall patient satisfaction with treatment and with life circumstances, stability of relationships, use of prescribed medication, employment outcomes, and use of illicit drugs.

Supported by a grant from the Department of Veterans' Affairs Health Services Research and Development Service, the Social and Independent Living Skills program is being investigated in a controlled clinical trial with random assignment of chronic schizophrenic patients to either social skills training or psychosocial occupational therapy, which is characterized as a creative and expressive intervention. All patients receive medication management by the same team of psychiatrists, who are blind to the psychosocial treatment condition, and clinical case management by advanced degree clinicians. Case management is provided to patients in the two treatment conditions in a manner that is congruent with the prevailing psychosocial treatment condition; thus, patients in the social skills training condition receive case management that uses behavioral and learning techniques already employed in the social skills training classes. This congruence allows for greater generalization of treatment effects and clearly defines case management activities. Patients in the occupational therapy condition—which focuses on expressive activities, encouragement of interpersonal relations, and affective communication and insight—receive a form of case management that employs these same techniques and processes.

While our data are preliminary, they appear to herald the value of combining skills training with assertive case management. Evidence supports the conclusion that *patients in the social skills training condition are able to acquire new knowledge and skills*. In the targeted skills areas of conversation, medication management, recreation, and symptom management, both groups start our treatment interventions at similar levels of knowledge and skill. Those in the skills-training condition have demonstrated significant increases in their levels of skill, while those in the occupational therapy condition have remained at the same levels of knowledge and skills.

There is evidence that *quality of life is significantly improved for individuals in the skills-training condition*. Analysis of data from the first twenty-five subjects in our study indicates that those individuals assigned to the skills-training condition enjoy significantly greater improvement in the Lehman Quality of Life Scale than do individuals assigned to the occupational therapy condition. For example, when individuals entered treatment with a high level of dissatisfaction with life as a whole, they improved to a greater extent in the skills-training condition. In addition, on the subscale that indexes their satisfaction with the "amount of fun" that they experience, those in the skills-training condition showed a significant improvement, while those in the occupational therapy condition remained the same or worsened slightly.

In the first year, *none of the subjects in either condition experienced a relapse*. Relapse, defined as an exacerbation of psychotic symptoms as measured by the BPRS, was below the often-cited rate of 40 percent or more of patients receiving medication and supportive services, and even below the rate of 20 percent cited for individuals receiving short-term skills training or behavioral family treatment (Hogarty and others, 1986). The determinants of this low rate may be related to the intensive and comprehensive character of both treatment conditions, the assertive case management approach, or the synergistic interaction of these interventions.

Summary and Future Directions

We are now at a point in the treatment and rehabilitation of individuals with chronic mental illnesses, such as schizophrenia, where intriguing questions can be addressed with regard to the relationships among different treatment approaches, systems of care, and the quality of life. These individuals require long-term, often lifelong, biobehavioral treatment and rehabilitation, with emphasis placed on the comprehensiveness and continuity of that care. Case management, social skills training, and pharmacotherapy have been shown to be effective components of comprehensive treatment programs.

We have been impressed by the need to target levels and types of care based on patients' functional status and needs. While the design of the current program requires that all patients enroll in the same basic core curriculum in social skills training, future efforts will be more sensitive to patients' values and directed toward a more precise coupling of functional assessment and rehabilitation planning.

Congruent with the early findings of Stein and Test (Test, 1991) and others, where patients decompensated after being withdrawn from assertive community treatment, some of our patients experienced depression after completing the intensive six-month phase of the program. This depression seems related to the notable contrast in their daily routines, with decreased levels of encouragement, reinforcement, and structure subsequent to the intensive phase.

We have found it useful to have psychiatrists link their medication dosage decisions to careful assessment of patients' symptoms and functioning. Structured instruments such as the BPRS have guided and improved our practice of targeting our pharmacological interventions to maximize beneficial properties of medications and minimize their side effects. The levels of participation of patients in the skills-training modules have also provided useful feedback to the prescribing psychiatrists, who are then apprised of the patients' under- or overmedication.

Social skills training has become a mainstay in the treatment and rehabilitation of chronically mentally ill individuals. Standardized curricula for skills training are becoming more widely used and will allow for broader replication of promising results with this population. In the coming years, treatment packages that are modularized for ready application will be more available so that the diverse needs of this population are met in a more clinically and cost-effective fashion.

Case management, while often described in the treatment of the chronically mentally ill, has suffered from a lack of precise definition. Many have written about the beneficial effects of case management services in enhancing continuity of care and availability of services. However, the variability of the interventions labeled as case management is striking. We should see greater efforts to clearly and precisely define models of case management according to the activities employed. We advocate the adoption of a clinically informed, rehabilitative approach in case management, fully integrated with the clinical services provided elsewhere in the treatment system. By building functional bridges that interconnect similar philosophies of treatment and rehabilitation across program settings and over time, we can better guide our interventions toward optimal outcomes at the levels of symptoms, disability, and handicap.

References

Allness, D. J., Knoedler, W. H., and Test, M. A. "The Dissemination and Impact of a Model Program in Process, 1972–1984." In L. I. Stein and M. A. Test (eds.), *The Training in Community Living Model: A Decade of Experience.* New Directions for Mental Health Services, no. 26. San Francisco: Jossey-Bass, 1985.

Benton, M. K., and Schroeder, H. E. "Social Skills Training with Schizophrenics: A Meta-Analytic Evaluation." *Psychological Assessment: Journal of Consulting and Clinical Psychology,* 1990, *58,* 741-747.

Corrigan, P. W., Liberman, R. P., and Engel, J. D. "From Noncompliance to Collaboration in the Treatment of Schizophrenia." *Hospital and Community Psychiatry,* 1990, *41* (11), 1203-1211.

Eckman, T. A., Liberman, R. P., Phipps, C. C., and Blair, K. E. "Teaching Medication Management Skills to Schizophrenic Patients." *Journal of Clinical Psychopharmacology,* 1990, *10,* 33-38.

Hogarty, G. E., Anderson, C. M., Reiss, D. J., Kornblith, S. J., Greenwald, D. P., Jarna, C. D., and Madonia, M. J. "Family Psychoeducation, Social Skills Training, and Maintenance Chemotherapy in the Aftercare Treatment of Schizophrenia." *Archives of General Psychiatry,* 1986, *43,* 633-642.

Kuehnel, T. G., and Liberman, R. P. "Functional Assessment." In R. P. Liberman (ed.), *Psychiatric Rehabilitation of Chronic Mental Patients.* Washington, D.C.: American Psychiatric Press, 1988.

Liberman, R. P. "Social Skills Training." In R. P. Liberman (ed.), *Psychiatric Rehabilitation of Chronic Mental Patients.* Washington, D.C.: American Psychiatric Press, 1988.

Liberman, R. P., Mueser, K. T., and Wallace, C. J. "Social Skills Training for Schizophrenic Individuals at Risk for Relapse." *American Journal of Psychiatry,* 1986, *143,* 523-526.

Liberman, R. P., Mueser, K. T., Wallace, C. J., Jacobs, H. E., Eckman, T. A., and Massel, H. U. "Training Skills in the Psychiatrically Disabled: Learning Coping and Competence." *Schizophrenia Bulletin,* 1986, *12,* 631-647.

Stein, L. I., and Test, M. A. "Alternatives to Mental Hospital Treatment. Part 1: Conceptual Model, Treatment Program, and Clinical Evaluation." *Archives of General Psychiatry,* 1980, *37,* 392-397.

Test, M. A. "Training in Community Living." In R. P. Liberman (ed.), *Handbook of Psychiatric Rehabilitation.* Elmsford, N.Y.: Pergamon, 1991.

Vaccaro, J. V., and Liberman, R. P. "Integrating Skills Training and Case Management for Chronic Schizophrenics in a Community Mental Health Center." In M. Bassi (ed.), *Nuovi percorsi dell'assistenza psichiatrica* [New approaches to psychiatric treatment]. Bologna, Italy: O.S.C., 1989.

Vaccaro, J. V., Liberman, R. P., and Roberts, L. J. "Schizophrenia: From Institutionalization to Community Re-Integration." In A. Kales, C. M. Pierce, and M. Greenblatt (eds.), *The Contemporary Mosaic of Psychiatry in Perspective.* New York: Springer-Verlag, 1991.

Vaccaro, J. V., Pitts, D. B., and Wallace, C. J. "Functional Assessment." In R. P. Liberman (ed.), *Handbook of Psychiatric Rehabilitation.* Elmsford, N.Y.: Pergamon, 1991.

Van Putten, T., and Marder, S. R. "Behavioral Toxicity of Antipsychotic Drugs." *Journal of Clinical Psychiatry,* 1987, *48* (supplement), 13-19.

Wallace, C. J. "Functional Assessment in Rehabilitation." *Schizophrenia Bulletin,* 1986, *12,* 604-630.

Wallace, C. J., Boone, S. E., Donahoe, C. P., and Foy, D. W. "The Chronically Mentally Ill Disabled: Independent Living Skills Training." In D. Barlow (ed.), *Clinical Handbook of Psychological Disorders.* New York: Guilford, 1985.

Witheridge, T. F. "The Assertive Community Treatment Worker and Its Implications for Professional Training." *Hospital and Community Psychiatry,* 1989, *40,* 620-624.

JEROME V. VACCARO, M.D., is assistant professor of psychiatry at the UCLA School of Medicine, assistant chief of the Rehabilitation Medicine Service at the Brentwood (Psychiatric) Division of the West Los Angeles VA Medical Center, medical director for the study reported in this article, and investigator at the UCLA Clinical Research Center for Schizophrenia and Psychiatric Rehabilitation.

ROBERT PAUL LIBERMAN, M.D., is professor of psychiatry at the UCLA School of Medicine, chief of the Rehabilitation Medicine Service at the Brentwood (Psychiatric) Division of the West Los Angeles VA Medical Center, principal investigator for the study reported in this article, and director of the UCLA Clinical Research Center for Schizophrenia and Psychiatric Rehabilitation.

CHARLES J. WALLACE, Ph.D., is director of research for the study reported in this article and chief of the Behavioral Assessment and Social Skills Laboratory in the UCLA Clinical Research Center for Schizophrenia and Psychiatric Rehabilitation.

GAYLA BLACKWELL, M.S.W., R.N., is chief of the Brentwood VA Social and Independent Living Skills program and project director for the study reported in this article.

By combining the therapeutic and rehabilitative effects of assertive community treatment, family psychoeducation, and the multifamily group, better use of an expanded social network yields a more coordinated clinical effort and an enhanced level of community adaptation for patients with chronic schizophrenia.

Family-Aided Assertive Community Treatment: A Comprehensive Rehabilitation and Intensive Case Management Approach for Persons with Schizophrenic Disorders

William R. McFarlane, Peter Stastny, Susan Deakins

Although there is still controversy about the ultimate wisdom of deinstitutionalization, states generally are continuing to implement this policy (Gralnick, 1985; Okin, 1985; Lamb, 1982; Minkoff, 1987). Hospital censuses continue to decline (New York State Office of Mental Health, 1988), and many state mental health administrations have embarked on major initiatives to develop treatment and rehabilitation capacity in local communities for the severely mentally ill. Among these initiatives, there is an increasing emphasis on psychiatric rehabilitation as a core element in the treatment philosophy and in the everyday practice of clinicians who deal with this population. The approach to rehabilitation described here brings together clinical and rehabilitative efforts in the patient's natural environment to achieve meaningful employment through education, guidance, and collaboration within a patient's family and among groups of families and patients.

We gratefully acknowledge the contributions to the development of this model made by the staffs of the participating clinics, Soundview-Throgs Neck Mental Health Center, New Rochelle Guidance Center, and Ulster County Mental Health Services, and by the project site directors, Peter Provet, Ph.D., Kathleen Moses, M.S.W., and Joann Gurian, M.S.W.

The resulting amalgam provides focused training in work and problem-solving skills in the context of a greatly expanded social support system.

Supported by federal and state grants, the Biosocial Treatment Research Division of the New York State Psychiatric Institute designed and evaluated a novel treatment and rehabilitation program for chronic schizophrenics. The program is served by public agencies and is based on two empirically validated approaches: Training in Community Living (TCL), also known as the Program of Assertive Community Treatment (PACT), and Psychoeducational (PE) or Behavioral Family Management. Comprehensive reviews of the studies supporting the efficacy of these approaches—in terms of reduced relapse and rehospitalization, improved social functioning, and enhanced quality of life—have recently been published (Test, 1992; Strachan, 1992). The aim of the present program development was to capitalize on the strengths and minimize the weaknesses of each of its constituent approaches.

Combining TCL and PE Multifamily Groups: A Rationale

The treatment strategies represented by TCL, on the one hand, and family psychoeducation and multifamily groups, on the other, appear to be solidly established as effective methods for reducing relapse and enhancing community functioning. However, each method contains a crucial limitation: TCL has not adequately addressed family participation in treatment, and the family approaches do not deal adequately with the rehabilitation needs of the severely mentally ill patient.

As a method that relies extensively on existing community resources and direct therapeutic support by teams of clinicians, TCL has shown a complicated relationship to the client's family and to the concept of building supportive networks. Initially, TCL promoted "constructive separation" of the patient from his or her family during crisis episodes. Further, patients were encouraged to live away from their families' homes and restrict their contacts with family members, who usually were not included in the treatment effort. As initially conceived, the TCL approach made extensive reference to the family literature of the 1950s, which emphasized pathogenetic characteristics of the family bond in schizophrenia (Ludwig and Farrelly, 1967). Recently, TCL proponents have made more of an effort to include family members, but not systematically and not as an integral part of the patient's rehabilitation.

In the case of family intervention approaches, wherein outcome is determined more by negative *patient* factors (for example, chronic medicational noncompliance, substance abuse, poor vocational achievement prior to onset of illness, and severely debilitating negative symptoms), family interaction and support, even if ideal, is less likely to positively affect the patient's course of rehabilitation. Our studies have consistently shown that approximately 10 percent of the sample patients suffered repeated relapses and rehospitalizations; that is, there were no observable effects from family intervention. Also, because the family models conform to an outpatient therapy profile, they rely on conventional vocational rehabilitation services. If these are refused by the patient or are not available, rehabilitation is much less likely to occur. Some families, though involved and motivated, may simply be too burdened to devote the necessary energy to the treatment and rehabilitation effort.

Thus, from these considerations, we came to the conclusion that a combination of TCL and the PE multifamily group might lead to enhanced outcomes, compared to TCL or psychoeducation alone, because each method compensates for crucial deficiencies in the other. Further, neither TCL nor psychoeducation significantly expands the patient's or the family's social network, whereas a multifamily group, by definition, does exactly that, thereby potentially adding an increment of efficacy. We term the combined approach Family-Aided Assertive Community Treatment (FACT). This approach fosters maximum possible coordination between all of the important people and social forces that influence a given patient. Although both of the source treatment models in FACT espouse and create continuity of care, each is deficient in bringing all of the components of the patient's treatment into one coordinated system.

FACT Study. The FACT research project began in 1987, sponsored by the New York State Office of Mental Health and the New York State Alliance for the Mentally Ill. The FACT project used a two-cell experimental design: one cell combined the TCL treatment method with PE multifamily group (FACT), and the other cell was TCL treatment with limited single-family crisis intervention (TCL). This design tested ongoing family participation in a multifamily group as a primary treatment factor.

The sample consists of seventy-two patients at three community mental health centers in New York state. Patients who met the following criteria were selected: diagnosis of DSM-III-R schizophrenia or schizophreniform and schizoaffective disorders, associated complicating factors (homelessness, treatment noncompliance, substance abuse, criminal charges, suicidality), family availability, and eighteen to forty-five years of age. Analysis of baseline psychiatric and demographic data indicated that no differences existed between cohorts.

Relapse rates after the first twelve months of treatment indicated that the FACT program had fewer relapses (22 percent) than the TCL-only program (40 percent). We have not included statistical analyses because this study is still underway. Preliminary analyses indicate that hospitalizations for the sample as a whole are reduced by over 50 percent from pretreatment levels. As with relapse, at twelve months FACT is superior to TCL alone in (1) number of patients employed at any job, whether full-time, part-time, in a sheltered workshop, or as a volunteer (37 percent versus 15.4 percent) and (2) competitive employment (16 percent versus 0 percent).

In summary, evidence now exists that (1) a multifamily group version of psychoeducation yields significantly fewer relapses than does the single-family form, (2) there is a significant increase in employment in both forms of PE family treatment and a trend toward superiority for the multi-family group format, and (3) FACT yields better vocational outcome than does TCL alone.

FACT as a Rehabilitation Approach

The FACT approach consists of interrelated elements, with unique aspects that include the PE multifamily group.

TCL Intervention. TCL is a comprehensive, biopsychosocial inter-vention designed to improve the community functioning of the severely mentally ill, thereby diminishing their reliance on inpatient care while improving their quality of life. TCL focuses on practical life concerns and assumes that the vast majority of mentally ill individuals can live satisfacto-rily outside the hospital with professional support and skills training. Derived from the TCL program in Madison, Wisconsin, and its extension, PACT, the efficacy of TCL has been well documented over the last two decades. TCL comprises six programmatic components (a detailed treat-ment manual of this approach is available on request):

Integration of the Patient's Life into the Community. As an alternative to hospitalization, TCL provides the patient with a viable support system in the community. This support calls for an assertive approach with consid-erable outreach and proactive monitoring in which TCL staff function as direct providers of individualized therapeutic and rehabilitation services, rather than as service brokers.

In Vivo Teaching of Coping and Problem-Solving Skills. To meet the de-mands of community life, patients must not only have adequate access to all material resources but also learn how to use them effectively. In addi-tion, problems of daily living and vocational adjustment arise frequently and require an array of problem-solving skills. As much as possible, the teaching of these skills takes place in vivo, that is, directly in the natural settings of the patients.

Prevention of Relapse and Crisis Intervention. The tasks of monitoring social stressors, such as life events or transitions, and responding imme-diately and assertively to them are essential to the prevention of relapse and require treatment team awareness of prodromal signs. Medication man-agement and monitoring is an integral feature of this approach and requires close collaboration with the prescribing psychiatrist, who is usually a mem-ber of the TCL team. The team is available on a twenty-four-hour basis to respond to client emergencies and is reachable by all concerned parties.

Graduated Increases in Patient Responsibilities. The TCL approach maintains a continuous rehabilitative stance in looking for opportunities to help
patients move in the direction of their established goals and independence.
An assertive but graduated approach is maintained to support clients in
their striving toward higher functional levels. However, we also recognize
that precipitous and premature advances can contribute to the resurgence
of prodromal symptoms and ultimately lead to a relapse. Therefore, an
increase in support, careful preparation, and symptom monitoring accompany any significant increase in functional demands.

Support and Education of Community Members. Community members,
especially the patients' families and employers, frequently react to patients'
behavior in ways not supportive of community tenure. The goal of the TCL
team is to aid these key community members by providing them with
ongoing support and guidance.

Team Approach. TCL is provided by an interdisciplinary team whose
members are known to all the team's clients and serve relatively inter-
changeable functions. The team functions within a tightly organized and
pragmatic structure, with an emphasis on goal-oriented treatment planning.
Daily schedules and staff assignments are based on client needs and staff
availability.

PE Multifamily Group Treatment. This unique component of the
FACT approach integrates the family into the ongoing treatment and rehabilitation work conducted by the clinicians. The component is focused on
patient vocational rehabilitation, stepwise functional progression, early crisis intervention, and relapse prevention; it is as coordinated as possible
with the team's work and plans. We encourage the expansion of families'
social networks by in-group cross-family problem solving and social support
and out-of-group socializing. The multifamily group treatment is briefly
described below (a detailed treatment manual of this approach is available
on request).

Initial Interventions: Engagement, Goal Setting, and Family Education.
The engagement and educational interventions begin with a minimum of
three engagement sessions, in which the patient's primary clinician meets
with the individual family unit, usually without the patient present (Anderson, Hogarty, and Reiss, 1986). These sessions are accompanied by separate
meetings with the patient. In carrying out rehabilitation, the essential starting point is goal setting, with the patient as the central focus. For both
philosophical and practical reasons, we emphasize the patients' perceived
desires for their vocational and social lives as the nuclei of work by both
the FACT team and the families in the multifamily group. Thus, the initial
and crucial step in each case is to get a sense of the patient's previous
work history and his or her interests either in continuing a career already
started or in changing directions. This step occurs in the initial sessions
held with the patient alone and in the joint patient-family sessions.

cohort of patients due to join the PE multifamily group for nine sessions, beginning in tandem with the PE work-lies. These meetings are classlike, in which the team teaches ow to set a goal, decide on the steps necessary for its achieve-ow to deal with barriers that might impede success (Miller, 1990). When five to eight families have completed the "joining" process, the FACT team conducts the educational workshop, again usually without patients. In this presentation, we also closely follow Anderson, Hogarty, and Reiss's (1986) format, except that we present the biomedical aspects of schizophrenia by showing a standardized videotape, and we have added new guidelines and other components specifically geared to the vocational rehabilitation phase.

The Ongoing PE Multifamily Group. Following the workshop, the first meeting of the PE multifamily group is held; its format includes a biweekly meeting schedule, each session one and one-half hours in length, leadership by two FACT clinicians, and participation by five to eight patients and their families. Patients are strongly encouraged to attend and actively participate.

The general therapeutic purpose of the multifamily group is the implementation of the family guidelines presented in the workshop. This implementation is pursued in phases that are timed according to the clinical condition of the patients and that largely utilize a group-based problem-solving method. The multifamily group problem-solving approach is adapted from Falloon and Liberman's (1983) single-family version. Families are taught to use this method in the multifamily group, as a group function. It is the core of the multifamily group approach and has become increasingly acceptable to families and remarkably effective.

The first phase of the therapeutic process concentrates on the problems experienced by the patients as they begin their reentries into the world outside the protected confines of the hospital or clinic. A central goal during this phase is prevention of relapse, which is achieved by limiting functional expectations and demands and reducing the level of stimulation and stress in the social environment. The multifamily group maintains remission by systematically applying the group problem-solving method to difficulties encountered in implementing the family guidelines and fostering recovery. The rehabilitation phase in FACT should be initiated only by patients who have achieved clinical stability by successfully completing this community reentry phase.

As patient stability increases, the multifamily group functions in a role unique among psychosocial rehabilitation models: It operates as an auxiliary of the in vivo vocational rehabilitation effort conducted by the clinical team. The central emphasis during this phase is the involvement of both the family and the group in helping each patient to begin a gradual, step-by-step resumption of responsibility and socializing. The clinicians continue to use group-based problem solving and brain storming to identify and develop jobs, and to help individual patients obtain job placement and to enrich their social lives.

Family-Based Goal Setting. Because this process inevitably involves some reduction or postponement of previously held vocational goals, and because those goals are often held as strongly by family members as they are by patients, the progress and outcomes of the goal-setting classes are reported to the multifamily group as a regular part of each session. These reports allow each family to express doubts and reservations, opinions, or support, so that the final result of goal setting is something that has been ratified by the patient's own family in the public arena of the multifamily group. Further, the other families in the group are aware of each patient's intentions, making the vocational progress of the group's patients the project of the entire group, which, in turn, helps to define a positive group identity. Reciprocally, the families' ideas, opinions, and information can be taken back to the goal-setting class and incorporated into patients' rehabilitation aims.

Creating a Compendium of Potential Jobs. After the group completes the goal-setting process, several group meetings are spent on developing a list of possible job opportunities among the members of the group's families and their extended kin. Potential jobs may be located in the homes or businesses of group members, in those of relatives and friends outside the group, or in their workplaces or those of their kin. In this way, patients can work at jobs with members of other families in the group or their extended kin. Jobs may also be located by group members through informal connections, chance encounters (for instance, seeing help-wanted signs), or deliberate inquiry and community advocacy. Ultimately, families, in collaboration with the team and local family advocacy associations, may create jobs for the patients through community action. In general, these jobs are potentially less stressful, since they are embedded within the social network of the multifamily group and involve social connections that are inherently more familiar to the patients. To a large degree, we have modeled this approach after the usual methods (networks and personal connections) by which a mentally healthy individual obtains a job or job leads (Roessler and Hiett, 1983; Vandergoot, 1976; Granovetter, 1974; Granovetter, 1979). Family members may be asked to gather additional information on job possibilities between meetings, but actual job development is usually carried out by the team clinicians.

Individualized Job Finding. After the completion of the job opportunity compendium, the vocational or social rehabilitation process for each patient is broken into sequential steps. The achievement of the next rehabilitative step, usually employment, is raised as a focus in the problem-solving portion of the multifamily group. The members of the group and their extended kin are polled for sources of jobs, job leads, and even possibilities for job development with specific reference to one particular patient in the group. In this brain-storming process, various ideas are generated from participants in the multifamily group. These suggestions are then reviewed by the patient and his or her family, and a final plan is developed. This step usually involves job preparation, job development, coaching, planning and problem solving, all carried out in the field by the FACT team. The results of these efforts are then reported back to the team during rounds, treatment planning, *and* during the next multifamily group. If necessary, the process is repeated if initial results are disappointing.

FACT in Action: A Case Study

The case of a twenty-three-year-old man illustrates the interaction between multifamily group and TCL interventions. Mark was in the midst of his first psychotic break when he joined the FACT project in 1988. He had become assaultive toward his mother and sister, was disruptive by shouting in public, and had refused medication. His family, while opposed to medication, was at their wit's end when they applied for treatment. Less than a month following his intake into the project, Mark threatened to kill his mother with a knife that he had been concealing, convinced that he was part of a white supremacist group aiming to rid the country of communists. This episode led to his first and only hospitalization, for two and one-half months, during which he was first given antipsychotic medication. He became less agitated and his psychosis remitted to the point that the family tolerated his return home.

Their acceptance was in part related to the beginning of multifamily group meetings while Mark was still an inpatient. As stipulated by his mother and reinforced by the FACT team and the multifamily group, a contract was negotiated for his release, which included medication, monitoring, and restriction against reading or even ordering incendiary and weapons-oriented literature. When a mercenary magazine arrived in the mail three months later, the mother reported this to the multifamily group and the ensuing problem solving enabled her to confront Mark about the magazine for the first time, with positive results. During this period FACT staff visited the client at home to assist with daily life skills and medication monitoring.

Upon recommendation of the team, he began to attend a day treatment program and shortly thereafter was evaluated for a vocational rehabilitation program at a sheltered workshop. An initial placement in a shoe factory was not successful, and FACT staff assisted Mark in securing a part-time job with the city sanitation department. The staff made regular visits to him at the job, when he returned to the sheltered workshop, and throughout a third work-trial with the city parks department. By that time the patient was assigned responsibility over his medication intake. His intermittent compliance raised concerns in the mother and prompted further problem solving in a multifamily group session. A number of life events ensued, including a move and the death of an aunt, throughout which Mark and his mother received extra support from the multifamily group and the FACT team.

For the past year Mark has remained actively involved in vocational rehabilitation without successful long-term placement in competitive employment. Family crises required attention in the multifamily group, while Mark expanded his social circle to include a number of substance abusers. He used his prescribed medication inconsistently and became overtly psychotic, requiring active psychiatric intervention. In spite of these setbacks, FACT staff continued to help him with job applications and two work-trials at a state-run betting parlor and a picture-framing workshop. At this time, he is working on his resume and preparing to attempt longer-term employment.

Conclusion

In an effort to capitalize on the specific advantages and efficacies of TCL, multifamily groups, and family psychoeducation, we have combined them into the comprehensive treatment system called FACT. Our aim is to make the multifamily group a task force, in which experts from various sectors of the patient's total network share experiences, information, and planning and create new ideas and options, especially in the area of vocational rehabilitation. The professional team's job is then to take these possibilities and attempt to realize them. The assumptions are that all aspects of the patient's network should be brought to bear on the effort toward employment and that expansion of that network through the business connections in a multifamily group can gain each patient access to a large pool of potential jobs and opportunities. This total process has contributed to the high employment rates achieved to date in our experimental clinical trial of the FACT approach.

References

Anderson, C. M., Hogarty, G. E., Bayer, T., and Needleman, R. "Expressed Emotion and Social Networks of Parents of Schizophrenic Patients." *British Journal of Psychiatry*, 1984, *144*, 247-255.

Anderson, C. M., Hogarty, G. E., and Reiss, D. J. *Schizophrenia and the Family*. New York: Guilford, 1986.

Berman, K. K. "Multiple Family Therapy: Its Possibilities in Preventing Readmission." *Mental Hygiene*, 1966, *50*, 367-370.

Bond, G. R. "An Economic Analysis of Psychosocial Rehabilitation." *Hospital and Community Psychiatry*, 1984, *35*, 356-362.

Bond, G. R., and Boyer, S. L. "Rehabilitation Programs and Outcomes." In J. A. Ciardiello and M. D. Bell (eds.), *Vocational Rehabilitation of Persons with Prolonged Psychiatric Disorders*. Baltimore, Md.: Johns Hopkins University Press, 1988.

Bond, G. R., Miller, L. D., Krumweid, R. D., and Ward, R. S. "Assertive Case Management in Three CMHCs: A Controlled Study." *Hospital and Community Psychiatry*, 1988, *39*, 411-418.

Brown, G. W., Birley, J.L.T., and Wing, J. K. "Influence of Family Life on the Course of Schizophrenic Disorders: A Replication." *British Journal of Psychiatry,* 1972, *121,* 241–258.

Doane, J. A., Falloon, I.R.H., Goldstein, M. J., and Mintz, J. "Parental Affective Style and the Treatment of Schizophrenia." *Archives of General Psychiatry,* 1985, *42,* 34–42.

Dozier, M., Harris, M., and Bergman, H. "Social Network Density and Rehospitalization Among Young Adult Patients." *Hospital and Community Psychiatry,* 1987, *38,* 61–64.

Falloon, I.R.H., and Liberman, R. P. "Behavioral Family Interventions in the Management of Chronic Schizophrenia." In W. R. McFarlane (ed.), *Family Therapy in Schizophrenia.* New York: Guilford, 1983.

Field, G., Allness, D., and Knoedler, W. H. "Application of the Training in Community Living Program to Rural Areas." *Journal of Community Psychology,* 1980, *8,* 9–15.

Garrison, V. "Support Systems of Schizophrenic and Non-Schizophrenic Puerto Rican Women in New York City." *Schizophrenia Bulletin,* 1978, *4,* 561–596.

Gralnick, A. "Build a Better State Hospital: Deinstitutionalization Has Failed." *Hospital and Community Psychiatry,* 1985, *36,* 738–741.

Granovetter, M. S. "The Strength of Weak Ties." *American Journal of Sociology,* 1973, *78,* 1360–1380.

Granovetter, M. S. *Getting a Job: A Study of Contacts and Careers.* Cambridge, Mass.: Harvard University Press, 1974.

Hammer, M., Makiesky-Barrow, S., and Gutwirth, L. "Social Networks and Schizophrenia." *Schizophrenia Bulletin,* 1978, *4,* 522–545.

Hogarty, G. E., Anderson, C. M., Reiss, D. J., Kornblith, S. J., Greenwald, D. P., Javna, C. D., and Madonia, M. J. "Psychoeducation, Social Skills Training and Maintenance Chemotherapy in the Aftercare Treatment of Schizophrenia." *Archives of General Psychiatry,* 1986, *43,* 633–642.

Hogarty, G. E., Anderson, C. M., Reiss, D. J., Kornblith, S. J., Greenwald, D. P., Ulrich, R. F., and Carter, M. "Family Psychoeducation, Social Skills Training, and Maintenance Chemotherapy in the Aftercare Treatment of Schizophrenia." *Archives of General Psychiatry,* 1991, *48,* 340–347.

Hogarty, G. E., McEvoy, J. P., Munetz, M., DiBarry, A. L., Bartone, P., Cather, R., Cooley, S. J., Ulrich, R. F., Carter, M., and Madonia, M. "Dose of Fluphenazine, Familial Expressed Emotion, and Outcome in Schizophrenia." *Archives of General Psychiatry,* 1988, *45,* 797–805.

Knoedler, W. H. "How the Training in Community Living Program Helps Patients Work." In L. I. Stein (ed.), *Community Support Systems for the Long-Term Patient.* New Directions for Mental Health Services, no. 2. San Francisco: Jossey-Bass, 1979.

Kopeikin, H. S., Marshall, V., and Goldstein, M. J. "Stages and Impact of Crisis-Oriented Family Therapy in the Aftercare of Acute Schizophrenia." In W. R. McFarlane (ed.), *Family Therapy in Schizophrenia.* New York: Guilford, 1983.

Lamb, H. R. *Treating the Long-Term Mentally Ill.* San Francisco: Jossey-Bass, 1982.

Lansky, M. R., Bley, C. R., McVey, G. G., and Botram, B. "Multiple Family Groups as Aftercare." *International Journal of Group Psychotherapy,* 1978, *29,* 211–224.

Leff, J. P., Kuipers, L., Berkowitz, R., Eberlein-Vries, R., and Sturgeon, D. "A Controlled Trial of Social Intervention in the Families of Schizophrenic Patients." *British Journal of Psychiatry,* 1982, *141,* 121–134.

Leff, J. P., and Vaughn, C. E. *Expressed Emotion in Families.* New York: Guilford, 1985.

Lipton, F. R., Cohen, C. I., Fischer, E., and Katz, S. E. "Schizophrenia: A Network Crisis." *Schizophrenia Bulletin,* 1981, *7,* 144–151.

Ludwig, A. M., and Farrelly, F. "The Weapons of Insanity." *American Journal of Psychotherapy,* 1967, *21,* 737–749.

Lukoff, D., Ventura, J., Liberman, R. P., and Nuechterlein, K. H. "Integrating Symptom Assessment into Psychiatric Rehabilitation." In R. P. Liberman (ed.), *Handbook of Psychiatric Rehabilitation.* Elmsford, N.Y.: Pergamon, 1992.

Lurie, A., and Ron, H. "Socialization Program as Part of Aftercare Planning." *General Psychiatric Association Journal*, 1972, *17*, 157-162.

Miller, S. *Goal-Setting: A Treatment Manual*. Unpublished manuscript, 1990.

New York State Office of Mental Health. *The Chartbook of Mental Health Information*. Albany: New York State Office of Mental Health, 1988.

Okin, R. L. "Expand the Community Care System: Deinstitutionalization Can Work." *Hospital and Community Psychiatry*, 1985, *36*, 742-745.

Olfson, M. "Assertive Community Treatment: An Evaluation of the Experimental Evidence." *Hospital and Community Psychiatry*, 1990, *41*, 634-641.

Pattison, E. M., Llama, R., and Hurd, G. "Social Network Mediation of Anxiety." *Psychiatric Annals*, 1979, *9*, 56-67.

Roessler, R. T., and Hiett, A. "Strategies for Increasing Employer Response to Job Development Surveys." *Rehabilitation Counseling Bulletin*, 1983, *26*, 368-370.

Sokolovsky, J., and Cohen, C. I. "Toward a Resolution of Methodological Dilemmas in Network Mapping." *Schizophrenia Bulletin*, 1981, *7*, 109-116.

Stein, L. I., and Ganser, L. J. "Wisconsin's System for Funding Mental Health Services." In J. A. Talbott (ed.), *Unified Mental Health Systems: Utopia Unrealized*. New Directions for Mental Health Services, no. 18. San Francisco: Jossey-Bass, 1983.

Stein, L. I., and Test, M. A. "Alternatives to Mental Hospital Treatment. Part 1: Conceptual Model, Treatment Program, and Clinical Evaluation." *Archives of General Psychiatry*, 1980a, *37*, 392-397.

Stein, L. I., and Test, M. A. "Alternatives to Mental Hospital Treatment. Part 3: Social Cost." *Archives of General Psychiatry*, 1980b, *37*, 409-412.

Stein, L. I., and Test, M. A. (eds.). *Alternatives to Mental Hospital Treatment*. New York: Plenum, 1978.

Strachan, A. "Family Management." In R. P. Liberman (ed.), *Handbook of Psychiatric Rehabilitation*. Elmsford, N.Y.: Pergamon, 1992.

Test, M. A. "Training in Community Living." In R. P. Liberman (ed.), *Handbook of Psychiatric Rehabilitation*. Elmsford, N.Y.: Pergamon, 1992.

Test, M. A., Knoedler, W. H., and Allness, D. J. "The Long-Term Treatment of Young Schizophrenics in a Community Support Program." In L. I. Stein and M. A. Test (eds.), *The Training in Community Living Model: A Decade of Experience*. New Directions for Mental Health Services, no. 26. San Francisco: Jossey-Bass, 1985.

Tolsdorf, C. C. "Social Networks, Support, and Coping: An Exploratory Study." *Family Process*, 1976, *15*, 407-417.

Vandergoot, D. V. "A Comparison of Two Mailing Approaches Attempting to Generate the Participation of Businessmen in Rehabilitation." *Rehabilitation Counseling Bulletin*, 1976, *20*, 73-75.

Vandergoot, D. V., Maiman-Reich, B., and Murphy, G. "Increasing the Motivation of Job Searchers." Unpublished manuscript, Human Resources Center, New York, 1983.

Vaughn, C. E., and Leff, J. P. "The Influence of Family and Social Factors on the Course of Psychiatric Illness: A Comparison of Schizophrenic and Depressed Neurotic Patients." *British Journal of Psychiatry*, 1976, *129*, 125-137.

Witheridge, T. F., and Dincin, J. "An Assertive Outreach Program in an Urban Setting." In L. I. Stein and M. A. Test (eds.), *The Training in Community Living Model: A Decade of Experience*. New Directions for Mental Health Services, no. 26. San Francisco: Jossey-Bass, 1985.

Worrall, J., and Vandergoot, D. V. "Additional Indicators of Non-Success: A Follow-up Report." *Rehabilitation Counseling Bulletin*, 1982, *26* (2), 88-93.

Zadny, J. J., and James, L. F. "Job Placement in State Vocational Rehabilitation Agencies: A Survey of Techniques." *Rehabilitation Counseling Bulletin*, 1979, *22* (4), 361-378.

WILLIAM R. MCFARLANE, M.D., is director of the Fellowship in Public Psychiatry and chief of the Biosocial Treatment Research Division at New York State Psychiatric Institute in New York City. He is associate clinical professor in the Department of Psychiatry of the College of Physicians and Surgeons at Columbia University.

PETER STASTNY, M.D., is senior clinical supervisor in the Biosocial Treatment Research Division and assistant clinical professor in psychiatry at Albert Einstein College of Medicine, Bronx, New York.

SUSAN DEAKINS, M.D., is senior clinical supervisor in the Biosocial Treatment Research Division and assistant clinical professor of psychiatry in the College of Physicians and Surgeons at Columbia University.

Rehabilitation of individuals with concomitant schizophrenia and stimulant abuse, once deemed futile, now seems feasible and promising.

Effectively Treating Stimulant-Abusing Schizophrenics: Mission Impossible?

Lisa J. Roberts, Andrew Shaner, Thad A. Eckman, Douglas E. Tucker, Jerome V. Vaccaro

Drug abuse among chronic psychiatric patients is widely recognized as a significant clinical and social problem and presents enormous challenges for clinicians, social service agencies, and health care systems (Ridgely, Goldman, and Talbott, 1986; Gorman, 1987; Cooper, Anglin, and Brown, 1989; Drake and Wallach, 1989). This problem is especially characteristic of schizophrenics, who abuse stimulants such as cocaine and amphetamine. Such dually diagnosed patients have probably existed since the original availability of d-amphetamine in 1936 (Davidoff and Rubenstein, 1939), but they have recently become a more prominent medical and social problem due to deinstitutionalization, the societal emergence of drug subcultures, and widespread homelessness. Epidemiological studies have reported a high rate of stimulant abuse among schizophrenics (McLellan and Druley, 1977; Richard, Liskow, and Perry, 1985) in both community and treatment settings. One third of schizophrenics admitted to the inpatient wards at the West Los Angeles Veterans Affairs (VA) Medical Center abuse cocaine (Wilkins, in press).

Stimulant-abusing schizophrenic patients are challenging and frustrating to treat. Both stimulant abuse and schizophrenia are chronic, severe, and presently incurable. When they occur together, each disorder often interferes with recognition and treatment of the other. Both patients and caregivers may ascribe symptoms entirely to substance abuse or to schizophrenia, thereby facilitating denial and interfering with effective treatment. Even when both disorders are recognized, integrated treatment may be precluded by parochial approaches to comorbidity. Mental health professionals may view stimulant abuse as an overwhelming, voluntary resistance to the treatment of schizophrenia, while addiction clinicians may view schizophrenia as too complex and strange to allow involvement in substance abuse treatments.

The reality seems to be that co-occurring stimulant abuse and psychotic disorders are deeply intertwined. Stimulant abuse may hasten the onset of schizophrenia (Mueser and others, 1990) and exacerbate its course by precipitating psychotic relapse (Richard, Liskow, and Perry, 1985), or by causing depression, anxiety, insomnia, or agitation (Alterman, Erdlen, McLellan, and Mann, 1980; Alterman and Erdlen, 1983; Yesavage and Zarcone, 1983). Stimulant abuse has also been associated with increased aggressiveness (Yesavage and Zarcone, 1983), increased rates of psychiatric hospitalization (Richard, Liskow, and Perry, 1985; Safer, 1987; Brady and others, 1990), and a tendency toward postpsychotic or secondary depression (Siris and others, 1988). Many clinicians believe that little can be done for these patients as long as they abuse stimulants. Likewise, schizophrenia may worsen concomitant stimulant abuse, as patients self-medicate depression, negative symptoms, or medication side effects (Siris and others, 1988; Schneier and Siris, 1987; Benson and David, 1986). Frequently, the net result is repeated cycles of emergency hospitalization for acute psychosis precipitated by drug abuse, followed by elopement and noncompliance when treatment fails to address the broad and interlocking array of clinical problems.

Given the problems associated with concomitant schizophrenia and stimulant abuse, it may seem paradoxical to say that stimulant-abusing schizophrenic patients have a better prognosis than do schizophrenics who do not abuse drugs. However, there are several reasons to believe that with effective treatment of stimulant abuse, the remaining symptoms of schizophrenia will be relatively mild. Dixon and others (1991) conducted a study that lends some support to this hypothesis. The study compared hospitalized substance-abusing schizophrenic patients to non-substance-abusing schizophrenics. At the time of admission, the severity of symptoms was the same in the two groups. However, at the time of discharge one month later, those who had abused substances had fewer positive and negative symptoms of schizophrenia. The authors suggested that better-prognosis schizophrenics have the social skills needed to obtain drugs. They concluded that when abstaining from drugs and treated appropriately, these patients are less symptomatic than poor-prognosis schizophrenics who do not abuse drugs. There are additional reasons to expect improved prognosis. First, each disorder may contribute to overall morbidity in an additive fashion. In other words, some patients who have severe overall illness may have mild schizophrenia complicated by stimulant abuse. Second, it is possible that in some vulnerable individuals, stimulants maintain a disorder that closely resembles schizophrenia. This implies that some patients who actually do not have schizophrenia may appear to have it because of stimulant abuse. Thus, among patients with similar levels of psychopathology and functional impairment, those who abuse stimulants may have a better prognosis for schizophrenia in the absence of substance abuse.

As of early 1990, only two published studies had examined the effectiveness of outpatient treatment for schizophrenic substance abusers in general, including some stimulant abusers (Hellerstein and Meehan, 1987; Kofoed, Kania, Walsh, and Atkinson, 1986). These studies prospectively followed for one year small cohorts of substance-abusing schizophrenic outpatients receiving specialized group therapy. Both studies found that patients who remained in treatment tended to abstain from substance use and had significantly fewer days of hospitalization than did patients who dropped out of treatment. The patients who remained in treatment also showed a reduced rate of hospitalization compared with their record prior to entering specialized treatment. Both treatment programs had high dropout rates (30 percent and 66 percent, respectively, after three months), and neither study obtained follow-up data on patients who dropped out, making it impossible to determine whether and to what extent a selection bias was operating.

The rationale for the development of our clinical program has been the "stress-vulnerability" model of illness in which various stressors and protective factors act on an underlying diathesis to disease expression. For example, it has been suggested that stimulants act as stressors on an underlying neurobiological vulnerability to schizophrenia. In response to stimulants, vulnerable individuals may develop psychosis more quickly, at lower doses, and for a longer period after the drug is stopped (Gold and Bowers, 1978; Post and Kopanda, 1976). Similarly, symptoms associated with schizophrenia can act as stressors or precipitants for stimulant abuse, as patients seek stimulants to relieve negative symptoms, neuroleptic side effects, depression, or social isolation. Medication, coping abilities, and social supports could serve as protective factors for individuals with either or both disorders. Inherent to this model is the assumption that both schizophrenia and stimulant abuse are responsive to stressors and protective factors that impinge on the disorders.

Dual Diagnosis Treatment Program

At the West Los Angeles Veterans Administration (VA) Medical Center and UCLA Department of Psychiatry, we have developed the Dual Diagnosis Treatment Program (DDTP), dedicated to the acute treatment and long-term rehabilitation of stimulant-abusing schizophrenics. Mental health and substance abuse clinicians and researchers joined in 1990 to form a multidisciplinary team that approaches patient care with a combination of pharmacological, psychoeducational, behavioral, and case management techniques. Our approach is based on comprehensive techniques of psychosocial treatment and rehabilitation of schizophrenia (Vaccaro and Liberman, 1989; Vaccaro, Liberman, Wallace, and Blackwell, this volume), adapted to meet the needs of stimulant-abusing schizophrenics. The new program aims to help patients establish and maintain community tenure. To achieve this goal the DDTP (1) combines acute inpatient treatment and long-term outpatient rehabilitation of both disorders in a single setting, (2) organizes clinicians into continuous treatment teams with long-term responsibility for a limited number of patients, (3) uses behavioral skills training to enhance social functioning and prevent relapse of both schizophrenic episodes and drug abuse, and (4) closely monitors drug abuse through self-report and urine testing.

Most patients enter the DDTP during an episode of acute psychosis or other crisis requiring hospitalization. Rather than merely resolve the immediate crisis, the program works to prevent future crises by teaching patients the specific information and skills that they need to prevent the relapse of active psychosis and stimulant abuse and to improve social functioning.

The DDTP treatment schedule includes the following groups: (1) relapse prevention module, (2) medication management module, (3) symptom management module, (4) psychoeducation group, (5) peer support group, (6) pre- and postweekend groups, (7) family group, (8) successful living group, (9) recreation/leisure module, (10) individual meetings with case manager, and (11) medication clinic. Twelve-step groups, based on the Alcoholics Anonymous model, have been modified to take into account the unique needs of dual diagnosis patients and have been integrated into this multifaceted treatment program (Minkoff, 1989).

DDTP is imbedded in a clinical research design that aims to evaluate the overall efficacy of the comprehensive program and the contributions of each of the major components to the overall outcomes of stimulant-abusing schizophrenics. Three conditions are compared: (1) DDTP that combines assertive case management and skills training, (2) customary VA care augmented by assertive case management, and (3) customary VA care. Assessments are conducted before treatment, after treatment, and during one year of follow-up, using a multilevel battery of biobehavioral instruments and interviews and urine toxicologies.

Social Skills Training. Guided by the stress-vulnerability model, we aim to protect stimulant-abusing schizophrenics from stress-induced relapse through enhanced coping skills and case management support. Behavioral self-management skills are taught through the use of a series of training modules whose practicality and efficacy have been demonstrated in a variety of settings (Eckman, Liberman, Phipps, and Blair, 1990; Hogarty and others, 1986; Liberman and Eckman, 1989; Liberman and others, 1986;

Wallace and Liberman, 1985; Wirshing, Eckman, Liberman, and Marder, 1991). Patients learn skills such as how to recognize warning signs of schizophrenic relapse (symptom management module), how to manage medication side effects (medication management module), and how to avoid illicit drugs and alcohol (relapse prevention module). Faculty at the UCLA Clinical Research Center have designed a training module specifically to teach schizophrenic patients the skills necessary to avoid and contain the use of cocaine and amphetamines (relapse prevention module). This module is based on the conceptualization of relapse proposed by Marlatt and Gordon (1985). The relapse prevention module educates patients about the risks and hazards of using drugs, helps them to identify precursors to drug relapse, and assists in the development of skills needed to cope with stress, negative emotions, and interpersonal conflict. The training procedures have been designed to compensate for the cognitive and social problem-solving deficits commonly found in schizophrenics and substance abusers.

Assertive Case Management. In providing social support via long-term individual case management, we have taken as a paradigm the Training in Community Living and Program for Assertive Community Treatment model, a successful program developed and evaluated by Stein and Test (1980). Multidisciplinary treatment teams (Torrey, 1986) headed by senior clinicians treat patients continuously, whether they are hospitalized or living in the community. Each team is responsible for addressing the needs of a specific group of patients, and each patient is assigned to a member of the continuous treatment team for individual case management (Harris and Bachrach, 1988). Each staff member has individual responsibility for eight to ten patients. Case managers help patients apply newly learned skills in real-life situations, working with family members, residential care home operators, and other natural support systems. Case management and skills training are integrated by training professional and paraprofessional staff members to deliver both services simultaneously and with high fidelity (Vaccaro and Liberman, 1989).

DDTP Case Studies

Our first case vignette demonstrates the efficacy of case management integrated with skills training in maintaining continuity of care and teaching the skills necessary to promote long-term progress:

> Harold had been repeatedly hospitalized for stimulant abuse and schizophrenia. A majority of these hospitalizations were involuntary, evoked by odd, inappropriate, or aggressive behaviors resulting from the delusions that "people from the dark side were after" him. Prior to his admission to DDTP, Harold would remain in treatment until he

received his monthly disability check. As soon as his money arrived, he would slip off the unit, contact a drug dealer, use the drugs that he had purchased, and return to the ward. Invariably, urine assays administered routinely on the ward would detect that he had used drugs, and in accordance with program policy, he would be discharged from the unit. To help Harold overcome this problem, his DDTP case manager arranged to accompany Harold when he picked up his check and deposited his funds. Together they created a budget and money management system. On one occasion, after selling drugs to an undercover police officer, Harold was arrested and sent to the local county jail. His case manager contacted the jail staff to inform them of Harold's prescribed medications and also to establish a plan to reinstitute treatment upon his release.

After returning from jail and resuming participation in the relapse prevention module and the symptom management module, Harold identified his personal "warning signs" of relapse for both substance use and schizophrenia. Based on past experiences, he realized that "bad or disappointing" news often led to his use of cocaine, which exacerbated his auditory hallucinations. Knowing that Harold had applied for a VA-service-connected pension, his case manager helped him develop a strategy to cope effectively with bad news. He practiced replacing self-defeating thoughts with positive statements and scheduled pleasant activities such as socializing with friends or going to a movie. His case manager created opportunities for Harold to practice role-playing his new skills and reinforced the use of a structured problem-solving method when potential obstacles arose. Weeks later, Harold's pension application was denied; however, he successfully implemented his relapse prevention plan and did not use drugs. Harold told his case manager that "by practicing 'thinking smart' I think I can stay clean and manage my schizophrenia better." With this mastery experience, his self-efficacy increased and he began to realize that with careful planning he could manage occasional setbacks while consolidating his gains.

The following case vignette illustrates the specific contribution that skills training can make in the rehabilitation of dual diagnosis patients.

Mark, a forty-year-old schizophrenic, was referred to DDTP after he spent his pension and disability checks on a cocaine binge that left him homeless, demoralized, and hallucinating. Cycles of cocaine binges, homelessness, and exacerbations of psychosis had resulted in eight hospitalizations during the previous three years. Most of these hospitalizations ended when Mark left the program against medical advice or without informing the staff of his departure. After precipitously leaving, he would immediately use cocaine. Several times, he pretended to have psychotic symptoms to obtain hospitalization after spending all of his money on cocaine. In a discharge summary, his inpatient psychiatrist wrote, "The patient is essentially malingering and uses the hospital as a place to stay after he spends his money on cocaine. His prognosis is exceptionally poor."

He entered the DDTP and completed the symptom management and relapse prevention skills-training modules. In the symptom management module, he learned how to identify and manage his personal warning signs of schizophrenic relapse, identified and learned specific techniques for coping with persistent symptoms, and learned strategies for avoiding illicit drugs and alcohol. In the relapse prevention module, he learned to identify his own personal, interpersonal, and situational determinants of drug use, and how to monitor and cope with urges to use drugs. He now lives in a board-and-care home and attends the DDTP outpatient clinic for medication management and continuation of training in the relapse prevention module. He plans to move to an apartment when he receives his certificate from the Department of Housing and Urban Development.

During the past year, Mark has not experienced a recurrence of psychotic symptoms but he has used cocaine twice. However, these drug relapses have differed markedly from prior relapses. Nearly every month for the preceding three years, Mark spent his entire monthly income of $700 on cocaine binges that left him psychotic and homeless and often led to hospitalization. The two drug relapses that occurred during the year after the skills-training intervention involved small amounts of cocaine. Although he had more money in his pocket, Mark stopped each episode after spending less than $50. He immediately reported both relapses to the treatment team, and neither relapse led to psychosis, homelessness, or hospitalization.

Credit Incentive Program

A behavioral incentive program is another important component of DDTP. Incentive programs are effective in increasing appropriate behaviors and decreasing or eliminating inappropriate behaviors on both substance abuse and psychiatric wards (Ayllon and Azrin, 1968; Liberman and others, 1977). Incentives have also been demonstrated to enhance attendance in day treatment programs for dual diagnosis patients (Carey, 1990). The DDTP has adapted a credit card system in which patients have ample opportunities to earn "credits" by demonstrating such behaviors as good personal hygiene, participation in groups, and adherence to medication regimens. These credits can be used to purchase lunch and personal items, to visit relatives and friends in a special outpatient lounge, or to attend recreational outings. Reinforcers such as food, a quiet and safe area to socialize, and the opportunity to be in a supportive treatment milieu are extremely powerful, since most of the patients are either homeless or live in low-income areas inundated with drugs and crime. The incentive system has significantly increased patients' attendance in treatment groups and individual case management sessions.

The following case vignette describes the effect that a token economy can have in shaping desired behaviors.

Bill had been homeless for over four years, and most of his hygiene skills had deteriorated. His exposure to the elements led to routine health problems, including lice infestations and skin rashes. Upon hospitalization, he refused to improve his personal hygiene. However, he observed that other patients who practiced good hygiene behaviors were praised by the staff and earned credits that enabled them to purchase a wide variety of items. Through the use of the incentive system, Bill became more motivated to bathe and use the medications prescribed to alleviate his lice and rashes.

Summary

The development of effective treatment programs for dual diagnosis patients is in its initial stages, hampered by a variety of clinical, theoretical, administrative, and even sociopolitical obstacles. These patients are difficult to engage and treat effectively using standard systems of care. The Dual Diagnosis Treatment Program at the Brentwood VA Hospital integrates treatment for both stimulant abuse and chronic psychosis within one comprehensive program, emphasizing continuous treatment teams, optimal pharmacological management, behavior-shaping strategies, skills-training techniques, and assertive case management. The combination of these treatment approaches within one program appears to have helped some patients in our preliminary, one-year experience. Future publications will describe results from controlled outcome comparisons of DDTP with customary VA care.

References

Alterman, A., and Erdlen, D. "Illicit Substance Use in Hospitalized Psychiatric Patients: Clinical Observations." *Journal of Psychiatric Treatment and Evaluations*, 1983, 5 (4), 377–380.

Alterman, A., Erdlen, R., McLellan, T., and Mann, S. "Problem Drinking in Hospitalized Schizophrenic Patients." *Addictive Behaviors*, 1980, 5 (3), 273–276.

Ayllon, T., and Azrin, N. H. *The Token Economy*. New York: Appleton-Century-Crofts, 1968.

Benson, J. I., and David, J. J. "Coffee Eating in Chronic Schizophrenic Patients." (Letter) *American Journal of Psychiatry*, 1986, 143 (7), 940–941.

Brady, K., Anton, R., Ballenger, J. C., Lydiard, R. B., Adinoff, B., and Selander, J. "Cocaine Abuse Among Schizophrenic Patients." *American Journal of Psychiatry*, 1990, 147 (9), 1164–1167.

Carey, K. B., and Carey, M. P. "Enhancing the Treatment Attendance of Mentally Ill Chemical Abusers." *Journal of Behavior Therapy and Experimental Psychiatry,* 1990, *21* (3), 205-209.

Cooper, L., Anglin, D., and Brown, V. "Multiple Diagnosis: Aspects and Issues in Substance Abuse Treatment." Unpublished White Paper for the State of California Department of Alcohol and Drug Programs, 1989.

Davidoff, E., and Rubenstein, E. C., Jr. "The Results of Eighteen Months of Benzedrine Sulfate Therapy in Psychiatry." *American Journal of Psychiatry,* 1939, *95* (4), 945-970.

Dixon, L., Haas, G., Weiden, P. J., Sweeney, J., and Frances, A. J. "Drug Abuse in Schizophrenic Patients: Clinical Correlates and Reasons for Use." *American Journal of Psychiatry,* 1991, *148* (2), 224-230.

Drake, R. E., and Wallach, M. A. "Substance Abuse Among the Chronic Mentally Ill." *Hospital and Community Psychiatry,* 1989, *40* (10), 1041-1046.

Eckman, T. A., Liberman, R. P., Phipps, C. C., and Blair, K. E. "Teaching Medication Management Skills to Schizophrenic Patients." *Journal of Clinical Psychopharmacology,* 1990, *10* (1), 33-38.

Gold, M. S., and Bowers, M. B. "Neurobiologic Vulnerability to Low Dose Amphetamine Psychosis." *American Journal of Psychiatry,* 1978, *135* (12), 1546-1548.

Gorman, C. "Bad Trips for the Doubly Troubled." *Time,* 1987, *130* (5), 58.

Harris, M., and Bachrach, L. L. (eds.). *Clinical Case Management.* New Directions for Mental Health Services, no. 40. San Francisco: Jossey-Bass, 1988.

Hellerstein, D., and Meehan, B. "Outpatient Group Therapy for Schizophrenic Substance Abusers." *American Journal of Psychiatry,* 1987, *144* (10), 1337-1339.

Hogarty, G. E., Anderson, C. M., Reiss, D. J., Kornblith, S. J., Greenwald, D. P., Javna, C. D., and Madonia, M. J. "Family Psychoeducation, Social Skills Training, and Maintenance Chemotherapy in the Aftercare Treatment of Schizophrenia." *Archives of General Psychiatry,* 1986, *43* (7), 633-642.

Kofoed, L., Kania, J., Walsh, T., and Atkinson, R. M. "Outpatient Treatment of Patients with Substance Abuse and Other Co-Existing Psychiatric Disorders." *American Journal of Psychiatry,* 1986, *143* (7), 867-872.

Liberman, R. P., and Eckman, T. A. "Dissemination of Skills Training Modules to Psychiatric Facilities: Overcoming Obstacles to the Utilization of a Rehabilitation Innovation." *British Journal of Psychiatry,* 1989, *155* (supplement 5), 117-122.

Liberman, R. P., Fearn, C. H., DeRisi, W. J., Roberts, J., and Carmona, M. "The Credit Incentive System: Motivating the Participation of Patients in a Day Hospital." *British Journal of Social and Clinical Psychology,* 1977, *16,* 85-94.

Liberman, R. P., Mueser, K. T., Wallace, C. J., Jacobs, H. E., Eckman, T. A., and Massel, H. K. "Training Skills in the Psychiatrically Disabled: Learning Coping and Competence." *Schizophrenia Bulletin,* 1986, *12* (4), 631-647.

McLellan, A. T., and Druley, K. A. "Non-Random Relation Between Drugs of Abuse and Psychiatric Diagnosis." *Journal of Psychiatric Research,* 1977, *13* (3), 179-184.

Marlatt, G. A., and Gordon, J. R. (eds.). *Relapse Prevention: Maintenance Strategies in Addictive Behavior Change.* New York: Guilford, 1985.

Minkoff, K. "An Integrated Treatment Model for Dual Diagnosis of Psychosis and Addiction." *Hospital and Community Psychiatry,* 1989, *40* (10), 1031-1036.

Mueser, K. T., Yarnold, P. R., Levinson, D. F., Singh, H., Bellack, S., Kee, K., Morrison, R. L., and Yadalam, K. G. "Prevalence of Substance Abuse in Schizophrenia: Demographic and Clinical Correlates." *Schizophrenia Bulletin,* 1990, *16* (1), 31-56.

Post, R. M., and Kopanda, F. T. "Cocaine, Kindling, and Psychosis." *American Journal of Psychiatry,* 1976, *133* (6), 627-634.

Richard, M. L., Liskow, B. I., and Perry, P. J. "Recent Psychostimulant Use in Hospitalized Schizophrenics." *Journal of Clinical Psychiatry,* 1985, *46* (3), 79-83.

Ridgely, M. S., Goldman, H. H., and Talbott, J. A. *Chronic Mentally Ill Young Adults with*

Substance Abuse Problems: A Review of Relevant Literature and Creation of a Research Agenda. Mental Health Policy Studies. Baltimore: University of Maryland School of Medicine, 1986.

Safer, D. J. "Substance Abuse by Young Adult Chronic Patients." *Hospital and Community Psychiatry,* 1987, *38* (5), 511-514.

Schneier, F. R., and Siris, S. G. "A Review of Psychoactive Substance Use and Abuse in Schizophrenia: Patterns of Drug Choice." *Journal of Nervous Mental Disease,* 1987, *175* (11), 641-652.

Siris, S. G., Kane, J. M., Frechen, K., Sellew, A. P., Mandeli, J., and Fasano-Dube, B. "Histories of Substance Abuse in Patients with Post-Psychotic Depressions." *Comprehensive Psychiatry,* 1988, *29* (6), 550-557.

Stein, L. I., and Test, M. A. "Alternatives to Mental Hospital Treatment. Part 1: Conceptual Model, Treatment Program, and Clinical Evaluation." *Archives of General Psychiatry,* 1980, *37* (4), 392-397.

Torrey, E. F. "Continuous Treatment Teams in the Care of the Chronically Mentally Ill." *Hospital and Community Psychiatry,* 1986, *37* (12), 1243-1247.

Vaccaro, J. V., and Liberman, R. P. "Integrating Skills Training and Case Management for Chronic Schizophrenics in a Community Mental Health Center." In M. Bassi (ed.), *Schizofrenia e cronicita* [Schizophrenia and chronicity]. Rome, Italy: CIC Edizione Internazionali, 1989.

Wallace, B. C. "Psychological and Environmental Determinants of Relapse in Crack Cocaine Smokers." *Journal of Substance Abuse Treatment,* 1989, *6,* 95-106.

Wallace, C. J., and Liberman, R. P. "Social Skills Training for Patients with Schizophrenia: A Controlled Clinical Trial." *Psychiatry Research,* 1985, *15* (3), 239-247.

Wilkins, J. N., Shaner, A. L., Patterson, C. M., Setoda, D., and Gorelick, D. "Discrepancies Among Patient Report, Clinical Assessment, and Urine Analysis in Psychiatric Patients During Inpatient Admission." *Psychopharmacology Bulletin,* in press.

Wirshing, W., Eckman, T. A., Liberman, R. P., and Marder, S. R. "Management of Risk of Relapse Through Skills Training of Chronic Schizophrenics." In C. A. Tamminga and S. C. Schulz (eds.), *Advances in Neuropsychiatry and Psychopharmacology.* Vol. 1: *Schizophrenia Research.* New York: Raven Press, 1991.

Yesavage, J., and Zarcone, V. "History of Drug Abuse and Dangerous Behavior in Inpatient Schizophrenics." *Journal of Clinical Psychiatry,* 1983, *44* (7), 259-261.

LISA J. ROBERTS, M.A., is coordinator of the Treatment of Schizophrenia and Stimulant Abuse research project and staff research assistant at the UCLA Clinical Research Center for Schizophrenia and Psychiatric Rehabilitation.

ANDREW SHANER, M.D., is chief of evaluations and admissions, VA Medical Center, West Los Angeles, Brentwood Division; assistant professor of psychiatry at UCLA; and principal investigator of the Treatment of Schizophrenia and Stimulant Abuse research project at the UCLA Clinical Research Center for Schizophrenia and Psychiatric Rehabilitation.

THAD A. ECKMAN, Ph.D., is program director of the Dual Diagnosis Treatment Program, VA Medical Center, West Los Angeles, Brentwood Division; research psychologist at UCLA; and project director of the Treatment of Schizophrenia and Stimulant Abuse research project at the UCLA Clinical Research Center for Schizophrenia and Psychiatric Rehabilitation.

DOUGLAS E. TUCKER, M.D., is medical director of the Dual Diagnosis Treatment Program, VA Medical Center, West Los Angeles, Brentwood Division; assistant clinical professor of psychiatry at UCLA; and co-investigator of the Treatment of Schizophrenia and Stimulant Abuse research project at the UCLA Clinical Research Center for Schizophrenia and Psychiatric Rehabilitation.

JEROME V. VACCARO, M.D., is assistant chief of Rehabilitation Medicine Service, VA Medical Center, West Los Angeles, Brentwood Division; assistant professor of psychiatry at UCLA; and co-investigator of the Treatment of Schizophrenia and Stimulant Abuse research project at the UCLA Clinical Research Center for Schizophrenia and Psychiatric Rehabilitation.

Institutionalized persons with a deteriorating form of schizophrenia that was refractory to neuroleptic medication were titrated downward in their haloperidol dose. Based on ratings of their clinical status, an optimal dose was reached that was an average 66 percent reduction from their initial levels. Patients then participated in a personalized, intensive behavior therapy program to remediate their extreme, persisting deficits and disturbances in behavior.

Optimal Drug and Behavior Therapy for Treatment-Refractory Institutionalized Schizophrenics

Timothy G. Kuehnel, Robert P. Liberman, Barringer D. Marshall, Jr., Linda Bowen

Despite innumerable positive reports on the efficacy of antipsychotic medication, there remains an enormous reservoir of persons with schizophrenia and other chronic psychoses who are refractory to this form of therapy. It has been estimated that upward of 500,000 chronically psychotic persons in the United States are relatively refractory to the array of antipsychotic drugs currently in use (Angrist and Schulz, 1990). Although a new generation of novel antipsychotic drugs promises to reduce the staggering scope of this public health problem, treatment-refractory patients will continue to fill state hospital beds, vegetate in community residences, and languish in abject poverty and homelessness on the streets of our major cities.

Treatment refractoriness has been defined operationally as "continuing psychotic symptoms with substantial functional disability and/or behavioral disturbances that persist in well-diagnosed persons with schizo-

We acknowledge the clinical contributions made by the interdisciplinary staff of the Camarillo-UCLA Clinical Research Unit, including Steve Green (recreation therapist), Joel Kelsch (social worker), Bill Green (unit supervisor), Jeffrey Hayden (psychometrist), and all fifteen nurses and psychiatric technicians of the unit. The administrative support of Frank Turley, Ph.D. (executive director of Camarillo State Hospital) and Sarla Gnanamuthu, M.D. (medical director of Camarillo State Hospital) was essential to the success of this work. The work was supported by a research contract from the California Department of Mental Health and Clinical Research Center Grant MH30911 from the National Institute of Mental Health.

phrenia despite reasonable and customary pharmacological and psychoso-cial treatment that has been provided continuously for at least two years" (Brenner and others, 1990, pp. 552–553). An alternative definition that probably captures a similar pool of patients requires "at least three periods of treatment in the preceding five years with neuroleptic agents from at least two different chemical classes, at dosages equivalent to or greater than 1,000 mg/day of chlorpromazine for a period of six weeks, each without significant symptomatic relief; and no period of good functioning within the preceding five years" (Kane, Honingfeld, Singer, and Meltzer, 1988, p. 478).

For the past two decades, the professional staff of the Camarillo–University of California, Los Angeles (UCLA), Clinical Research Unit at Camarillo State Hospital have conducted treatment research on persons with refractory schizophrenia. Because pharmacological agents are never prescribed, ingested, or metabolized in a socioenvironmental vacuum, the Clinical Research Unit has emphasized both psychosocial and pharma-cotherapeutic approaches in its treatment research (Liberman, Wallace, Teigen, and Davis, 1974; Liberman, McCann, and Wallace, 1976; Liberman, Marshall, and Burke, 1981; Wong, Slama, and Liberman, 1985; Massel, Corrigan, Liberman, and Milan, 1991). In this chapter, as the clinical research team of the unit, we describe the highly structured, behavior therapy programs used with treatment-refractory patients, and we summa-rize a study that has aimed to determine the optimal doses of antipsychotic medication and types of behavior therapy for these patients.

The Clinical Research Unit

An eleven-bed, coeducational unit located at a state hospital serving the Southern California area, the Clinical Research Unit (CRU) functions with a staff of fifteen licensed nurses and psychiatric technicians, a psychiatrist, a social worker, two psychologists, a research assistant, and a rehabilitation therapist. In addition, consultants to the unit include psychiatrists and psychologists from the UCLA faculty who are experts in neuropsychology, behavioral assessment and treatment, and psychopharmacology. Adjacent to the CRU are laboratories for assessments of psychophysiological, behav-ioral, cognitive, and neuropsychological functions. A close liaison connects the CRU with the psychopharmacology laboratory at the UCLA-Brentwood Veterans Affairs (VA) Hospital.

Core Behavioral Assessment and Treatment System. Essential to behavior therapy are repeated and reliable measurements of psychopathol-ogy, self-care and personal hygiene skills, social interaction, participation in recreational activities, and incident, interval, and time-sampling record-ing of individual behavioral assets, deficits, and deviances. Data from these thousands of assessments each day are summarized and graphed by the night shift using a personal computer. These summarized data are then used by the professional multidisciplinary team to guide its clinical decision making, as well as to provide feedback to patients at regularly scheduled meetings. Core behavior therapy programs are utilized to reduce or control aberrant behavior that serves as a barrier to community adaptation, as well as to develop or strengthen patients' functional skills.

A *credit incentive system* or token economy is used to provide motivation for patients who are typically anhedonic and amotivated and/or have difficulty learning. Immediate reinforcement for patients' appropriate and adaptive behavior is provided in the form of points and social reinforcement. A limited number of intolerable behaviors such as aggression, property destruction, and theft result in loss of points, which is termed a *response cost* procedure. Points can be exchanged for privileges, special activities, or tangible reinforcers throughout the day.

Brief *time-out from positive reinforcement* is utilized immediately following any act of assault or property destruction. Ordinarily, this practice is conducted in a "quiet area" designated by lines on the floor in a remote corner of the ward, but, in the absence of a patient's cooperation, a barren "quiet room" may be used. Withdrawal of attention, termed *extinction,* is employed for less serious aberrant behaviors, such as teasing and verbal aggression.

A *meal or eating program* stresses the acquisition and maintenance of appropriate, safe eating skills and social behavior and discourages inappropriate behaviors, such as wolfing down large bites of food and stealing food from peers.

Appropriate *hygiene, grooming, and living area maintenance skills* are encouraged through supervision and training, including use of verbal and visual prompts and shaping procedures if necessary. Daily programs include bathing, grooming, and dressing, toothbrushing, and room cleanup. *Appropriate appearance* throughout the day is accomplished by requiring patients to meet specified criteria during all credit exchanges.

Rehabilitation therapy is used to increase patients' functional skills in the areas of self-management of medication, conversational skills, and appropriate use of leisure time. Patients receive points, social reinforcement, and tangible reinforcement for active on-task behavior and nondisruptive behavior throughout and at the conclusion of these rehabilitation sessions.

While these core programs alone might be considered "intensive" behavior therapy interventions in many settings, at the CRU additional, individualized treatments for targeted behaviors unresponsive to the core programs are utilized. During the past twenty years, a wide array of disturbing behaviors were targeted for customized and effective intervention, including inappropriate sexual behavior, polydipsia, screaming and temper tantrums, social skills deficits, poor nutritional intake, incoherence and mumbling, self-injury, and suicidal attempts.

**Optimizing Neuroleptic Drug Therapy for Refractory Schizophren-
ics.** Because they have not responded optimally to customary dosage regimens of antipsychotic medication, treatment-refractory schizophrenics are often prescribed increasingly higher doses in search of a means of controlling their psychotic symptoms and disturbing, sometimes intolerable behaviors. Often, these high doses are pushed at the behest of anxious and helpless nursing staff who seek chemical restraint of dangerous or bizarre patients. Recent studies have found that the therapeutic index of neuroleptics is much narrower than previously believed (Baldessarini, Cohen, and Teicher, 1988; Van Putten, Marder, and Mintz, 1987). There is now evidence that some patients may actually appear treatment-resistant because their high doses and plasma levels of neuroleptic drug are producing behavioral toxicity and neurological side effects that mimic psychiatric symptoms or interfere with functional engagement in the psychosocial milieu (Van Putten and others, 1990, 1991).

To determine whether treatment-refractory schizophrenic patients might show an improved "benefit-risk ratio" when treated with lower doses of neuroleptic, a study was conducted on the CRU that systematically titrated patients' haloperidol doses downward from initially high levels to the point of optimal therapeutic response. Optimal response was operationalized as the lowest dose compatible with control of positive and negative symptoms and of behavioral disturbances while concurrently producing a minimum of side effects. Clinical response was monitored with a battery of assessment instruments, including the Brief Psychiatric Rating Scale as expanded by faculty at the UCLA Clinical Research Center for Schizophrenia and Psychiatric Rehabilitation, Target Symptom Scales, and measures of side effects, especially akathisia, extrapyramidal symptoms, and dyskinesias.

Thirteen treatment-refractory persons with schizophrenia (ten males and three females), meeting the criteria articulated earlier in this chapter, were transferred to the CRU on dosages of haloperidol ranging between 50 and 80 mg per day. Patients who were at the time concurrently receiving augmenting or adjunctive drugs (for example, lithium, benzodiazepines, or carbamazepine) had them gradually discontinued, without apparent detriment. After a ten-week baseline, each patient's haloperidol dosage was systematically reduced—on a double-blind basis—to 35, 20, 15, 10, 5, and 0 mg daily dosages. Decrements in dosage occurred every five weeks. Scheduled reductions in dosages were accomplished until each patient was judged clinically "much worse" by consensus of a seven-member, interdisciplinary treatment team using the Clinical Global Impressions Scale, which was rated by integrating observations of ward behavior, self-care, and psychopathology. When any patient reached the point deemed much worse by consensus of the treatment team, he or she was withdrawn from the dosage reduction phase and the next higher dosage was defined as the "optimal" treatment. Staff and patients alike were "blind" to the dosage reduction schedule.

The initial mean dosage of haloperidol for the thirteen patients in the study was 63 mg per day, and the final mean dosage at the "optimal" level was 22 mg per day. This yielded a 66 percent reduction in dosage on the average for all thirteen patients. Ten of the patients achieved daily haloperidol dosages of 20 mg per day or less. One patient was able to tolerate reduction to 0 mg (receiving a placebo for his daily medications) for two months, but he subsequently experienced a schizoaffective relapse and had to be returned to a moderate dose of maintenance neuroleptic and lithium. In only this case and one other was the clinical deterioration marked by exacerbation of characteristic psychotic symptoms; in the other case, the patient had a catatonic reaction. The remaining patients who survived dosage reduction experienced forms of clinical deterioration noted by the emergence of behavioral disturbances such as self-injurious and assaultive behaviors.

In 70 percent of the patients, the optimal haloperidol dosage was associated with a plasma level of haloperidol that fell within the "therapeutic window" of 5 to 12 ng/ml, which has been previously reported in treatment-responsive schizophrenic patients (Van Putten and others, 1991). Neither tardive dyskinesia nor the severity of psychopathology—whether for positive or negative psychotic symptoms—significantly changed from baseline to optimal dosage levels of haloperidol; however, the patients' scores on the measures of neurological side effects did show significant improvement with the decremental dosage titration. Both akathisia and extrapyramidal symptoms were reduced markedly, yielding a significant improvement in the overall benefit-risk ratio for the patients in the study.

After stabilization on the optimal, or lowest effective, dose, patients' Clinical Global Impressions Scale scores reflected some degree of improvement in eight of the eleven patients who completed the full protocol. Perhaps because of fewer side effects, patients' levels of participation in ward activities and self-care efforts improved. Nursing staff rated the patients as more actively involved and more alert and reported overall improvement in their clinical status. Notably, one measure of central nervous system information processing—the Span of Apprehension Test— discriminated the patients who could tolerate substantial dosage reduction from those who could not. The few patients with poor information processing appeared to need high doses of maintenance antipsychotic medication, which replicates a similar finding with a different cohort of patients at the Brentwood VA Hospital in Los Angeles (Asarnow and others, 1988).

Efficacy of Behavior Therapy at Optimal Neuroleptic Dose: A Case Study of Didi, the "Screamer"

It was expected that patients would become more responsive to intensive and individualized behavior therapy after stabilizing on a lower dose of haloperidol that was congruent with a better benefit-risk ratio. While the overall study findings on this point have not yet been fully analyzed, enough information is available to conclude that some, but not all, patients did show remarkably favorable responses to behavior therapy. Following a functional assessment of each patient's behavioral assets, deficits, and deviances—as well as a behavioral analysis of environmental antecedents and consequences of target symptoms—we developed highly structured behavior therapy programs for each of the patients who reached optimal dosage reduction of their haloperidol. The following case study illustrates a positive response to intensive and individualized behavior therapy.

Didi was a thirty-seven-year-old single female, who had been almost continuously hospitalized for chronic, paranoid schizophrenia since the age of thirteen. At the time of her transfer to the CRU to participate in the study of haloperidol reduction and behavior therapy, she was regressed, highly delusional, and extraordinarily disruptive and aggressive. She met the criteria for treatment refractoriness, operationalized as persisting psychotic symptoms, functional deficits, and behavioral disturbances, despite many years of continuous neuroleptic treatment.

She isolated herself much of the time in the female bathroom, hiding from staff and peers, primarily because she was frightened that someone was going to kill her or harm her in some way. Delusions of reference included her belief that people were talking about her and laughing at her. She would scream obscenities and incomprehensible threats for hours at a time, literally driving staff and fellow patients to distraction and ear plugs. Subsequent to shouting these beliefs, she would frequently strike or attempt to strike peers or staff who she believed were saying these things.

Somatic delusions included the belief that she has been dead or was dead. She also believed that her organs and her bones were destroyed by the handling that she had received when people tried to control her behavior. She would stand nude for hours about the unit, and if clothing was put on her she would strip again and rip the clothing apart. Attempting to screen her from view of the other patients would similarly result in her throwing the screen at peers or staff. She was obviously frightened at all times. She was socially isolated, apathetic, agitated, and her self-care skills were very poor. For example, she was indifferent to her personal hygiene and she refused to use pads or tampons to manage her menses.

She entered the drug reduction phase of the study on 65 mg per day of haloperidol. Her dose was systematically reduced every five weeks to 15 mg per day without signs of clinical worsening. Unit staff and other patients exercised tremendous patience with her throughout the drug reduction phase in spite of her continued personal deficits, screaming, aggression, and denudativeness. During the five months of decremental drug titration, the core behavioral programs used on the CRU did not reduce the intensity or frequency of Didi's negative behaviors.

An analysis of the antecedents of Didi's agitated screaming episodes, which frequently escalated to property destruction and assaultive behavior, was conducted and revealed the following triggering events: (1) She would become upset following requests or when demands were placed upon her, for example, when she was asked to clean up her room. She particularly did not like to be hurried. (2) When she received the attention of another and that attention ended or even momentarily turned away from her, she would get tense and begin shouting. (3) She would focus on someone else's conversation that was not directed at her and then perceive it as being directed at her. She would then begin to say in a whiny voice, "You're bothering me. They're bothering me." This would progress to a sustained scream. (4) Peers teasing her (real or imagined) and people touching her, particularly men, almost always precipitated screaming or aggression. Physical manifestations that occurred prior to full-blown screaming episodes included rapid single-arm rubbing, rapid stomping of feet, eyes widening as if surprised, and running up the hallway, often with a piece of clothing that she swung in an effort to strike someone.

Didi's idiosyncratic target symptoms and problem behaviors were defined by staff as screaming, stripping, and noncompliance with staff directions. A variety of interventions was designed and implemented in sequence, as follows:

1. Progressive muscle relaxation was tried as a method that Didi could use to calm herself down when she was becoming agitated. Unfortunately, she became more paranoid and tense when trying to learn the relaxation steps, since she equated tension reduction with loss of control and verbalized sexual mistreatment themes relative to previous periods in her life when she felt abused. After one week of attempting to train her in progressive relaxation, she refused to participate.

2. When Didi or staff noticed that she was becoming agitated, she was asked if she would like to relax in a soft chair in the CRU social worker's office and listen to soft music until she was calm. This intervention proved somewhat successful in delaying her agitations but did not decrease the overall frequency, duration, or intensity of these events.

3. Paradoxical interventions such as instructing her to scream were briefly tried to no avail.

4. A differential reinforcement of other behavior modification procedure was attempted in which Didi would receive "special reinforcers," such as brief walks off the unit with a staff member of her choice, for not becoming agitated for varying periods of time. This was only partially successful in that Didi would agree to the program and the screaming would be curtailed until shortly before she was to receive the reinforcer. The bursts of screaming just prior to the walks appeared to be more intense and of longer duration than were her customary episodes, so this procedure was discontinued.

5. Since Didi's acting-out behaviors were thought at least in part to be due to her anxiety stemming from her delusions and from her extreme social anxiety that precluded any chance of reality-testing her delusional misperceptions, a program of social skills training was instituted. Three to five times a day, five days per week, Didi received social skills training. These sessions averaged fifteen minutes in duration. During each session, Didi was given choices of the topic of the session, location of the session, when the session was to begin, with whom the session would be, what music would be played in the background, what she would eat or drink, and what materials or games would be used. We purposely built in these choices because we wanted her to gain experiences of feeling in control of her daily life. These sessions appeared to be enjoyable to her. She showed moderate gains in knowledge and skill in the areas of initiating and maintaining conversations; unfortunately, these social skill improvements did not produce any noticeable decline in her behavioral disturbances.

We still thought that the strategy of inducing relaxation would serve to reduce her level of overstimulation, preclude acts of aggression, and give others a period of peace and quiet. Thus, a "required relaxation" program, based on the work of Webster and Azrin (1972), was developed and implemented following approval by the hospital's Human Rights Committee.

First, to increase positive interactions and reinforcement, Didi was encouraged to request conservational sessions with staff members anytime that she wished. At these times, staff would take her for a brief walk and interact casually and warmly with her. Second, when Didi was becoming agitated (chasing others, threatening, rubbing her arm rapidly, repeatedly stating "I'm not Didi," or rapidly stomping her feet with her torso swaying), she was offered a choice of required relaxation or brief counseling with a walk. Third, for denudative behavior, agitation, assault, property destruction, or screaming, required relaxation was implemented.

Relaxation was defined as lying prone on a mat, still (no movement except eyes, eyelids, fingers, chestwall, or toes), and quiet (no vocalization) for five consecutive minutes initially and ten minutes for subsequent implementations of the procedures on the same day. Each time that target disturbing behaviors were emitted, Didi was given verbal instruction and requested to comply voluntarily. Any resistance or movement after lying prone resulted in application of manual guidance by staff to contain her until she met the criteria for relaxation. As she began to comply with instructions, staff gradually eased the manual guidance until it was no longer necessary. At the point that manual guidance was withdrawn and she was quiet, the timer was set for the five- or ten-minute interval. The timer was restarted at zero each time she failed to meet the behavioral criteria for relaxation. As can be seen in the behavioral graph shown in Figure 6.1, the number of incidents per day of screaming, assaults, and property destruction rapidly decreased by over 80 percent across the nearly twelve-month period.

Figure 6.1. Behavioral Graph of Didi's Required Relaxation Program

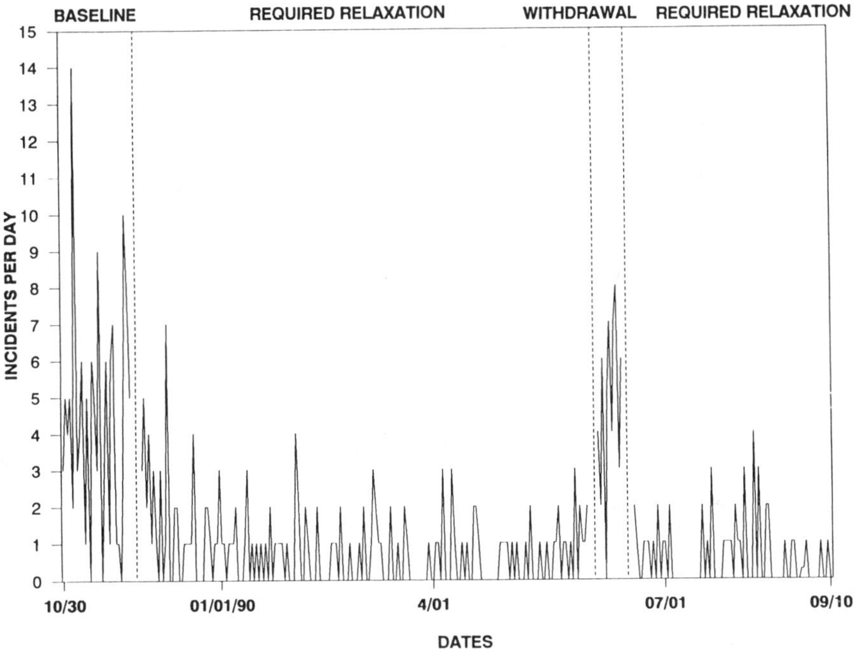

To ascertain the causal relationship between the required relaxation program and her behavioral improvement, a period wherein the program was withdrawn was introduced as an experimental within-subject control, after the program had been in operation for approximately six months. This withdrawal resulted in a rapid reacceleration of each of her disturbing targeted behaviors, so the required relaxation was again implemented after eight days. The required relaxation program immediately controlled target behaviors and was implemented until Didi was transferred back to her previous hospital unit. Follow-up indicated that Didi's incidents of screaming, assaultiveness, and property destruction were occurring at a somewhat higher rate than when she was on the CRU; however, the behavior therapy program is used sporadically by staff on her current unit, resulting in behavior that is still markedly better than when she was initially transferred to the research program.

Conclusion

Through an empirical, trial-and-error approach, behavior therapy programs, individualized according to a thorough functional assessment of each patient's deficits and disturbances, can result in meaningful improvements in apparently treatment-refractory patients. In the case of Didi, not only was her level of comfort increased but the quality of life of her fellow patients and caregiving staff was also raised. While effective behavior therapy requires a well-trained staff capable of frequent behavioral monitoring and consistent application of interventions and contingencies of reinforcement, such treatment does not require higher staff-patient ratios (Paul and Lentz, 1977).

Although some behavior analysts have argued that all dysfunctional behaviors serve a communicative function and can be replaced by adaptive behaviors that achieve for the individual those reinforcers served by the deviance (LaVigna, Willis, and Donnelan, 1989), the case of Didi highlights the importance of utilizing interventions that can decelerate disruptive behaviors while concomitantly offering opportunities to learn social and personal skills (Cipani, 1990; Liberman and Wong, 1984). Didi certainly benefited from efforts to teach her social and relationship skills; however, her most clinically disruptive problems were not adequately controlled until the direct, required relaxation program was implemented.

Our successful experience with dosage reduction of haloperidol in the treatment of refractory schizophrenics replicates and extends the findings of others who have studied dosage reduction with persistently psychotic outpatients (Faraone and others, 1989; Leblanc, Cormier, Gagne, and Vaillancourt, 1989). Lower neuroleptic dosages result in substantially reduced side effects and an enhanced benefit-risk ratio, which remove barriers to psychiatric rehabilitation. While most treatment-refractory schizophrenic patients may require sustained neuroleptic drug therapy, the dosages can often be vastly lower with significantly reduced exposure to the hazards and toxicity of high-dosage neuroleptic therapy. In addition, effective, individualized behavior therapy programs can prevent the creeping escalations of neuroleptic drug dosing that often result from the misguided efforts of clinicians under pressure to do something "therapeutic" for otherwise refractory patients.

References

Angrist, B., and Schulz, S. C. *The Neuroleptic-Nonresponsive Patient.* Washington, D.C.: American Psychiatric Press, 1990.

Asarnow, R. F., Marder, S. R., Mintz, J., Van Putten, T., and Zimmerman, K. "Differential Effects of Low and Conventional Doses of Fluphenazine on Schizophrenic Outpatients with Good or Poor Information Processing Abilities." *Archives of General Psychiatry,* 1988, *45,* 822–826.

Baldessarini, R. J., Cohen, B. M., and Teicher, M. H. "Significance of Neuroleptic Dose and Plasma Level in the Pharmacological Treatment of Psychoses." *Archives of General Psychiatry,* 1988, *45,* 79–91.

Brenner, H. D., Dencker, S. J., Goldstein, M. J., Hubbard, J. W., Keegan, D. L., Kruger, G., Kulhanek, F., Liberman, R. P., Malm, U., and Midha, K. K. "Defining Treatment Refractoriness in Schizophrenia." *Schizophrenia Bulletin,* 1990, *16,* 551–561.

Cipani, E. "The Communicative Function Hypothesis: An Operant Behavior Perspective." *Journal of Behavior Therapy and Experimental Psychiatry,* 1990, *21,* 239–247.

Faraone, S. V., Green, A. I., Brown, W., Yin, P., and Tsuang, M. T. "Neuroleptic Dose Reduction in Persistently Psychotic Patients." *Hospital and Community Psychiatry,* 1989, *40,* 1193–1195.

Kane, J., Honingfeld, G., Singer, J., and Meltzer, H. Y. "Clozapine for the Treatment-Resistant Schizophrenic." *Archives of General Psychiatry,* 1988, *45,* 789–796.

LaVigna, G. W., Willis, T. J., and Donnelan, A. M. "The Role of Positive Programming in Behavioral Treatment." In E. Cipani (ed.), *The Treatment of Severe Behavior Disorders: Behavior Analysis Approaches.* Washington, D.C.: American Association of Mental Retardation, 1989.

Leblanc, G., Cormier, H. J., Gagne, M. A., and Vaillancourt, S. "Effects of Neuroleptic Reduction in Schizophrenic Outpatients Receiving High Doses." Paper presented at the annual meetings of the American Psychiatric Association, May 1989.

Liberman, R. P., Marshall, B. D., and Burke, K. "Drug and Environmental Interventions for Aggressive Psychiatric Patients." In R. B. Stuart (ed.), *Control of Violence.* New York: Brunner/Mazel, 1981.

Liberman, R. P., McCann, M. J., and Wallace, C. J. "Generalization of Behaviour Therapy with Psychotics." *British Journal of Psychiatry,* 1976, *129,* 490–496.

Liberman, R. P., Wallace, C. J., Teigen, J., and Davis, J. "Interventions with Psychotics." In K. S. Calhoun, H. E. Adams, and E. M. Mitchell (eds.), *Innovative Treatment Methods in Psychopathology.* New York: Wiley, 1974.

Liberman, R. P., and Wong, S. E. "Behavioral Analysis and Therapy Related to Seclusion and Restraint." In K. Tardiff (ed.), *The Psychiatric Uses of Seclusion and Restraint.* Washington, D.C.: American Psychiatric Press, 1984.

Massel, H. K., Corrigan, P. W., Liberman, R. P., and Milan, M. "Conversation Skills Training for Thought-Disordered Schizophrenic Patients Through Attention-Focusing." *Psychiatry Research,* 1991, *38,* 51–61.

Paul, G. L., and Lentz, R. *Psychosocial Treatment of the Chronic Mental Patient.* Cambridge, Mass.: Harvard University Press, 1977.

Van Putten, T., Marder, S. R., and Mintz, J. "The Therapeutic Index of Haloperidol in Newly Admitted Schizophrenic Patients." *Psychopharmacology Bulletin,* 1987, *23,* 201–207.

Van Putten, T., Marder, S. R., Wirshing, W. C., Aravagiri, M., and Chabert, N. "Neuroleptic Plasma Levels." *Schizophrenia Bulletin,* 1991, *17,* 197–216.

Van Putten, T., Marder, S. R., Wirshing, W. C., and Midha, K. K. "Neuroleptic Plasma Levels in Treatment-Resistant Schizophrenic Patients." In B. Angrist and S. C. Schulz (eds.), *The Neuroleptic Non-Responsive Patient.* Washington, D.C.: American Psychiatric Press, 1990.

Webster, D. R., and Azrin, N. H. "Required for Relaxation: A Method for Inhibiting Agitated-Disruptive Behavior of Retardates." *Behaviour Research and Therapy,* 1973, *11,* 67–78.

Wong, S. E., Slama, K., and Liberman, R. P. "Behavioral Analysis and Therapy for Aggressive Psychiatric and Developmentally Disabled Patients." In L. Roth (ed.), *Clinical Treatment of the Violent Person.* New York: Guilford, 1985.

TIMOTHY G. KUEHNEL, Ph.D., is assistant research psychologist at the UCLA School of Medicine and staff psychologist at the Camarillo-UCLA Clinical Research Unit at Camarillo State Hospital, where he oversees the behavior therapy programs.

ROBERT PAUL LIBERMAN, M.D., is professor of psychiatry at the UCLA School of Medicine and director of the Camarillo-UCLA Clinical Research Unit, which he founded in 1970. He also directs the Clinical Research Center for Schizophrenia and Psychiatric Rehabilitation, which has performance sites at Camarillo State Hospital, Brentwood VA Hospital, UCLA Neuropsychiatric Institute and Hospital, UCLA Department of Psychology, and USC Department of Psychology.

BARRINGER D. MARSHALL, Jr., M.D., is assistant clinical professor of psychiatry at UCLA School of Medicine and clinical director and supervisor of the Camarillo-UCLA Clinical Research Unit.

LINDA BOWEN, Ph.D., is staff psychologist at the UCLA Department of Psychiatry and coordinator of research at the Camarillo-UCLA Clinical Research Unit.

Chronicity in serious mental disorders emanates from deficient ecological resources interacting with vulnerable individuals. Rehabilitation can succeed if an integrated and individualized approach is augmented by appropriate ecological supports.

Ecological Vocational Rehabilitation

J. P. Dauwalder, H. Hoffmann

A major shortcoming of rehabilitation approaches for the seriously mentally disabled is the prevailing attribution of patients' difficulties to themselves. While the aim of rehabilitation programs is to improve patients' skills and abilities to fulfill social roles, these programs rarely explore the obstacles and stressors present in the patients' environments. By exploring the person-environment "fit" within an ecological context, chronicity will be seen as maintained by inappropriate coping strategies of significant others as well as adverse situational constraints.

The following description of a typical case illustrates our approach. A. H., a forty-eight-year-old man, has been in psychiatric treatment since the age of twenty-nine. His clinical diagnosis is chronic schizophrenia (disorganized type). Even during his premorbid young adulthood, communication difficulties at work were reported. During a seven-year period, he worked at five different places. While living abroad for two years he lost contact with his family and former friends. Upon his return, he decompensated rapidly and was hospitalized for the first time. Despite repeated efforts by several employers, he systematically lost all jobs during the next fifteen years. The causes were always the same: Feeling overwhelmed, he got tense and nervous and finally provoked arguments with his superiors. For three years he lived in a sheltered home, working there as gardener. When he even lost this sheltered workplace, he was referred to our industrial rehabilitation unit.

Careful assessment of his instrumental abilities showed a performance level of about 50 percent of a normal worker. Main problems were identified in his social behavior with co-workers and superiors. Whereas social skills training proved inefficient, the patient was progressively integrated into our community-based ambulatory aftercare setting, which offers case management by a continuous treatment team. In this setting he got a "secondary" social network through regular contacts with caregivers and other former patients in the community. His slowly growing confidence in social relations was mainly reinforced by the availability of a drop-in facility called the *round table*. After ten months of vocational training in our rehabilitation unit, we found an appropriate ecological work "niche" for him in a print factory.

At present, he continues working half-time, lives independently together with two other former patients, and regularly visits our ambulatory aftercare setting. In the print factory, he and his immediate superiors and co-workers get regular support and consultation by the case manager, which is important to maintaining his job.

The progressive social withdrawal of this patient, observed for years before his admission to our services, was due not only to his psychopathology or inappropriate behavior but also to his lack of a socially supportive network and transitional ecobehavioral environment. His poor problem-solving abilities resulted in repeated failure: Whenever he got a job, he lost it.

There is now sufficient clinical and scientific evidence that carefully orchestrated social support of the patient's environment greatly enhances the effectiveness of rehabilitation programs (Falloon, 1985; Leff, 1987; Hogarty and Anderson, 1987; Angermeyer and Klusmann, 1989; Falloon, Hahlweg, and Tarrier, 1990). Usually, such intervention programs focus on the patient's family. Our experience suggests the added benefits of systematically including all other significant persons (for example, landlords or co-workers) from the social network of a patient.

For many chronic patients there exists only a minimal or no natural social network. In the case of A. H. we therefore had to build up a secondary social network in our ambulatory aftercare setting, in which the continuous treatment team facilitated communication and cooperation between all significant persons and coordinated all therapeutic steps (Hoffmann and Pia, 1990). In our perspective this approach was necessary to break the vicious cycle described above. Although his deficiencies in social behavior could not be fully remediated, he gradually acquired more social and leisure activities.

The final step in vocational rehabilitation, then, was to find an ecological niche, where superiors and co-workers were willing to cooperate with the continuous treatment team, which offered reliable support.

Training Facilities in the Natural Environment

Work contributes a unique and meaningful element to the rehabilitation process. No other activity can completely replace it. Work promotes social integration, development of identity, and self-confidence and makes social contacts and relationships possible. For a selected group of chronically mentally ill patients, intensive vocational training in specialized industrial rehabilitation units over one to two years has succeeded in promoting 25 to 45 percent of cases to competitive work (see, for example, Haerlin, 1985; Hubschmid and Aebi, 1986; Steinhart and Terhorst, 1988; Rudas, 1990). However, because this kind of training is appropriate only for a limited number of chronic patients, dropout rates of up to 40 percent within the first six months of such programs have been observed. Successful patients usually show better social skills at work and have shorter periods of previous unemployment and higher expectations for future employment (Ciompi, Dauwalder, and Ague, 1979). Another limitation comes from the socioeconomic context: Unemployment rates above 2 percent may seriously hamper access to competitive work, while unemployment rates above 6 percent may render competitive jobs almost inaccessible for the mentally ill (Morgan and Cheadle, 1975).

To cope with such adverse contexts, recent initiatives to create self-help firms that provide work for former psychiatric patients have proved to be successful (Seyfried, 1990). These work sites are indeed community based, but they have the disadvantage of releasing employers from the need to make jobs available to mentally disabled persons. This leads to segregation instead of integration, and the ghetto of chronic patients is shifted from the mental hospital into the community.

In general, psychiatry has not undertaken sufficient efforts to assimilate chronic patients into society and its labor market. Bond's (1990) metanalysis of twenty-four controlled studies suggests that rehabilitation programs succeed modestly in placing patients into jobs, but they fail to prepare these patients for future competitive employment outside the programs. On the other side, attempts to adapt workplaces in business, trade, and industry to the needs of chronic patients have so far been made only rarely. Vocational rehabilitation efforts over the past eight years in different Swiss cities have shown that it is possible to unite companies in the effort of establishing vocational training places in free enterprise. But it is up to professionals in rehabilitation to contact the employers and to find a common language. Collaboration with these companies produces encouraging results when the immediate superiors and the co-workers are well informed and get sufficient support from professionals.

An Integrated Vocational Rehabilitation Program

Our program addresses the needs of the mentally disabled who have not worked continuously for at least twelve months and have no organic or addictive disease. The aim of the program is to achieve optimal vocational and social rehabilitation and to stabilize the chronic patient at a higher level of functioning. The complete program has five phases with continuous ecobehavioral assessments. Continuous assessments give us important information about the ongoing process in order to make decisions on further steps within the program. The five phases are designed as follows:

Tryout. The two-week tryout phase in our rehabilitation unit offers opportunities for the patient to become familiar with different fields and demands of work. Our rehabilitation unit offers fifteen places for training in fields such as electronics, metalwork, and assembly tasks. The team consists of two full-time rehabilitation specialists and a social worker, a psychologist, and two psychiatrists, all part-time. During the tryout phase, the team gets a clinical grasp of the assets, resources, and deficits of the patient. At this time the first assessment is performed in order to establish a baseline. The results and personal impressions are discussed in a meeting, where all significant persons for a given patient participate. They clarify if the program meets the needs of the patient and if there are enough resources and sufficient predictors for a favorable outcome. These questions are important for reducing the dropout rate. If there are doubts about a patient's readiness for intensive vocational training, we might recommend reassignment to one of our time-unlimited sheltered workshops.

Rehabilitation Unit. For a maximum period of six months, the patient next receives vocational training in our rehabilitation unit. During this period, the first series of social skills training is offered. Communication, social competence, and problem-solving strategies are taught. Modules of symptom management, medication management, and job-interviewing skills are included. Furthermore, psychoeducational information on the nature of mental illness is given to relatives and future co-workers. Significant others are invited to join a group of relatives for all subsequent phases. According to the clinical course and periodic ecobehavioral assessments, the ongoing program is readjusted as necessary.

Training in Enterprise. In order to reduce the ghettolike situation of earlier rehabilitation workplaces, we offer "natural" training places, created in several business, trade, and industrial companies. While these places meet the patients' needs and interests, they also must be consistent with efficient running of the enterprise. Within the company, the places for training are decentralized to avoid a rehabilitation workshop atmosphere. These places supplement each company's normal employee rolls.

The places for training in enterprise are time-limited for each patient, from six to a maximum of eighteen months. For each participating company we offer a service package, including psychoeducational meetings for co-workers and immediate superiors, where we give information about schizophrenia and try to reduce prejudices and build up a collaborative atmosphere. Furthermore, our mobile rehabilitation team maintains case management, with two rehabilitation specialists regularly visiting the companies and giving support to the patients and to their superiors and co-workers. This continuous support has proved to be very important for the success of training in private enterprise. In case of problems, the company knows where to get help. If repeated efforts of problem solving at a work site fail, we take the patient back into our unit, whereby the patient returns twice a week to our unit for a second series of social skills training.

Integration. Lasting a maximum of six months, this phase is used for competitive job finding. If a patient's performance and interest and the company's satisfaction are congruent, a regular and permanent position in the firm may be offered. If not, another competitive job is sought with the help of the mobile rehabilitation team and the social worker. Similar to the company that participates in the training enterprise, the definitive employer is integrated into the rehabilitation process.

Aftercare. In the first month at a new job, but also later, psychosocial crises frequently occur. Superiors often try to hold onto a patient with too much patience and effort, until they are exhausted and give up. The long-term case management by our mobile rehabilitation team offers crisis intervention aimed at preventing the loss of the job.

Conclusion

Following the shift in psychiatric rehabilitative endeavors from institutional to community-based settings, the future of rehabilitation for chronic patients is in integrative, well-coordinated sociopsychiatric networks. In our program, the resources of natural environments are integrated into a new system-ecological perspective. Natural social and supportive networks encourage chronic psychiatric patients and significant others, within and outside of work site environments, to learn to adapt mutually. The potential of ecological systems for self-organization and absorption of disturbances might facilitate more rapid rehabilitation, beyond the customary negative expectations of professionals. Furthermore, stable, natural work environments for psychiatric patients, whatever their particular problems, may have preventive effects, such as earlier recognition of risks for relapse. Finally, patients and their relatives will suffer less from the still-prevailing social stigma attached to mental illness.

Hogarty and Anderson (1987) have shown that the combination of psychoeducative family therapy, social skills training, and maintenance medication can drastically reduce risks of relapse in schizophrenia. By analogy, we think that vocational training in private enterprise, including psychoeducation and support not only of relatives but also of relevant others at the work sites, delivered with continuous case management by a mobile rehabilitation team and with individualized social skills training, can minimize chronicity and accelerate progress in rehabilitation.

References

Andreasen, N. C. "The Diagnosis of Schizophrenia." *Schizophrenia Bulletin*, 1987, *13*, 9-22.

Angermeyer, M. C., and Klusmann, D. (eds.). *Soziales netzwerk. Ein neues könzept für die psychiatrie* [Social network: A new concept for psychiatry]. Berlin, Germany: Springer-Verlag, 1989.

Anthony, W. A., and Jansen, M. A. "Predicting the Vocational Capacity of the Chronically Mentally Ill: Research and Policy Implications." *American Psychologist*, 1984, *39*, 537-544.

Bachrach, L. "Assessment of Outcomes in Community Support Systems: Results, Problems, and Limitations." *Schizophrenia Bulletin*, 1982, *8*, 39-61.

Bachrach, L., and Lamb, R. H. "What Have We Learned from Deinstitutionalization?" *Psychiatric Annals*, 1989, *19*, 12-21.

Bond, G. R. "Vocational Rehabilitation." In R. P. Liberman (ed.), *Handbook of Psychiatric Rehabilitation*. Elmsford, N.Y.: Pergamon, 1991.

Brenner, H. D., Kraemer, S., Hermanutz, M., and Hodel, B. "Cognitive Treatment in Schizophrenia." In E. R. Straube and K. Hahlweg (eds.), *Schizophrenia: Concepts, Vulnerability, and Intervention*. Berlin, Germany: Springer-Verlag, 1990.

Carpenter, W. T., Heinrichs, D. W., and Alphs, L. D. "Treatment of Negative Symptoms." *Schizophrenia Bulletin*, 1985, *11*, 440-452.

Ciompi, L., Ague, C., and Dauwalder, J. P. "Ein Forschungsprogramm zur Rehabilitation psychisch Kranker [A research program for psychiatric rehabilitation]. II. Querschnittuntersuchung einer Population von chronischen Spitalpatienten. [Research on a cross-section of a population of chronically hospitalized patients]." *Nervenarzt*, 1978, *49*, 232-238.

Ciompi, L., Dauwalder, J. P., and Ague, C. "Ein Forschungsprogramm zur Rehabilitation psychisch Kranker [A research program for psychiatric rehabilitation]. III. Längsschnittuntersuchung zum Rehabilitationserfolg und zur Prognostik [Longitudinal research into rehabilitation success and prognosis]." *Nervenarzt*, 1979, *50*, 366-378.

Crow, T. J. "The Two-Syndrome Concept: Origins and Current Status." *Schizophrenia Bulletin*, 1985, *11*, 471-485.

Falloon, I.R.H. *Family Management of Schizophrenia*. Baltimore, Md.: Johns Hopkins University Press, 1985.

Falloon, I.R.H., Hahlweg, K., and Tarrier, N. "Family Intervention in the Community Management of Schizophrenia: Methods and Results." In E. R. Straube and K. Hahlweg (eds.), *Schizophrenia: Concepts, Vulnerability, and Intervention*. Berlin, Germany: Springer-Verlag, 1990.

Freeman, H., Fryers, T., and Henderson, J. *Mental Health Services in Europe: 10 Years On*. Geneva, Switzerland: World Health Organization, 1985.

Gleick, J. *Chaos—die Ordnung des Universums*. Munich, Germany: Droemer-Knaur, 1987.

Haerlin, C. H. "Arbeitstherapie—Berufliches Training—Arbeitsvermittlung am Biespiel des Beruflichen Trainingszentrums in Wiesloch [Work therapy—professional training—job placement in a professional work training center in Wiesloch]." In. G. Bosch and C. Kulnekampff (eds.), *Komplementäre Dienste—Wohnen und Arbeiten* [Complementary services—living and working]. Aktion Psyche, Tagungsberichte Band 11 [Conference proceedings vol. 2]. Cologne, Germany: Rheinland-Verlag, 1985.

Haken, H. *Advanced Synergetics*. Berlin, Germany: Springer-Verlag, 1987.

Hersen, M., and Barlow, D. H. *Single-Case Experimental Designs: Strategies for Studying Behavior Change*. Elmsford, N.Y.: Pergamon, 1976.

Hoffmann, H., and Pia, D. "Zur langfristigen Rehabilitation sozialpsychiatrischer Patienten." In L. Ciompi and H. P. Dauwalder (eds.), *Zeit und Psychiatrie. Sozialpsychiatrische Perspektiven*. Bern, Switzerland: Huber, 1990.

Hogarty, G. E., and Anderson, C. M. "A Controlled Study of Family Therapy, Social Skills Training, and Maintenance Chemotherapy in the Aftercare Treatment of Schizophrenic

Patients: Preliminary Effects on Relapse and Expressed Emotion at One Year." In J. S. Strauss, W. Boeker, and H. D. Brenner (eds.), *Psychosocial Treatment of Schizophrenia.* Toronto, Ontario, Canada: Huber, 1987.

Huber, G. "Das Konzept substratnaher Basissymptome und seine Bedeutung für Theorie und Therapie schizophrener Erkrankungen" [Theory and therapy for schizophrenic patients]. *Nervenarzt,* 1983, *54,* 23-32.

Hubschmid, T., and Aebi, E. "Vocational Rehabilitation of Psychiatric Long-Stay Patients: A Catamnestic Study." *Social Psychiatry,* 1986, *21,* 152-157.

Leff, J. P. "Changing the Family Environment of Schizophrenic Patients." In J. S. Strauss, W. Boeker, and H. D. Brenner (eds.), *Psychosocial Treatment of Schizophrenia.* Toronto, Ontario, Canada: Huber, 1987.

Liberman, R. P., and Evans, C. "Behavioural Rehabilitation for Chronic Mental Patients." *Journal of Psychopharmacology,* 1985, *5* (3), 8-14.

Liberman, R. P., Jacobs, H. E., Boone, S. E., Foy, D. W., Danahoe, C. P., Falloon, I.R.H., Blackwell, G., and Wallace, C. J. "Skills Training for the Community Adaption of Schizophrenics." In J. S. Strauss, W. Boeker, and H. D. Brenner (eds.), *Psychosocial Treatment of Schizophrenia.* Toronto, Ontario, Canada: Huber, 1987.

Liberman, R. P., Mueser, K. T., Wallace, C. J., Jacobs, H. E., Eckman, T. A., and Massel, H. K. "Training Skills in the Psychiatrically Disabled: Learning Coping and Competence." In E. R. Straube and K. Hahlweg (eds.), *Schizophrenia: Concepts, Vulnerability, and Intervention.* Berlin, Germany: Springer-Verlag, 1990.

Matson, J. "Behavior Modification Procedures for Training Chronically Institutionalized Schizophrenics." In M. Hersen, R. Eisler, and R. Miller (eds.), *Progress in Behavior Modification.* Vol. 9. San Diego, Calif.: Academic Press, 1980.

Minkoff, K. "Beyond Deinstitutionalization: A New Ideology for the Postinstitutional Era." *Hospital and Community Psychiatry,* 1987, *38,* 945-950.

Morgan, R., and Cheadle, A. J. "Unemployment Impedes Resettlement." *Social Psychiatry,* 1975, *10,* 63-67.

Morrison, R., and Bellack, A. "Social Functioning of Schizophrenic Patients: Clinical and Research Issues." *Schizophrenia Bulletin,* 1987, *13,* 715-725.

Rothbaum, R., Weisz, J., and Snyder, S. "Changing the World and Changing the Self: A Two-Process Model of Perceived Control." *Journal of Personality and Social Psychology,* 1982, *42,* 5-37.

Rudas, S. "Vocational Rehabilitation of Persons with Mental Illness in a Specialized Facility: Findings of a Study." *Rehabilitation,* 1990, *29,* 90-93.

Seyfried, E. "New Types of Work for Mental Patients." *Psychiatric Praxis,* 1990, *17,* 71-77.

Spring, B., Lemon, M., and Fergeson, P. "Vulnerabilities of Schizophrenia: Information-Processing Markers." In E. R. Straube and K. Hahlweg (eds.), *Schizophrenia: Concepts, Vulnerability, and Intervention.* Berlin, Germany: Springer-Verlag, 1990.

Steinhart, T., and Terhorst, B. "The Work Therapy Workshop as Part of a Psychiatric Care System: Its Contribution Towards Integrating Medical, Vocational, and Social Rehabilitation." *Rehabilitation,* 1988, *27,* 152-159.

Thomas, R. (ed.). *Kinetic Logic: A Boolean Approach to the Analysis of Complex Regulatory Systems.* Berlin, Germany: Springer-Verlag, 1979.

Thurm, I., and Haefner, H. "Perceived Vulnerability, Relapse, Risk, and Coping in Schizophrenia: An Explorative Study." *European Archives of Psychiatry and Neurological Sciences,* 1987, *237,* 46-53.

Wing, J. "Psychosocial Factors Affecting the Long-Term Course of Schizophrenia." In J. S. Strauss, W. Boeker, and H. D. Brenner (eds.), *Psychosocial Treatment of Schizophrenia.* Toronto, Ontario, Canada: Huber, 1987.

Zubin, J. "Suiting Therapeutic Intervention to the Scientific Models of Aetiology." *British Journal of Psychiatry,* 1989, *155* (5), 9-14.

J. P. DAUWALDER, Ph.D., is professor of clinical psychology at the University of Lausanne, Switzerland. He was formerly associated with the Social Psychiatric Clinic of the University of Bern, Switzerland.

H. HOFFMANN, M.D., is associate professor of psychiatry at the Social Psychiatric Clinic of the University of Bern, Switzerland, where he directs the clinical operations of the ecological vocational rehabilitation program described in this chapter.

By implementing intervention strategies to help psychiatrically disabled persons choose, get, and keep jobs, supported employment can become a successful element in psychiatric rehabilitation.

Choose-Get-Keep: A Psychiatric Rehabilitation Approach to Supported Employment

Karen S. Danley, Ken Sciarappa, Kim MacDonald-Wilson

Employment in competitive jobs is frequently desired, but seldom secured by people with psychiatric disabilities (Anthony, Farkas, and Cohen, 1990; Anthony, Cohen, and Danley, 1988; Unger and Anthony, 1984; Rogers, Walsh, Danley, and Smith, 1991). A metanalysis of vocational rehabilitation programs—designed to enhance clients' work skills, adjustment, hardening, job search, and placement—found them consistently, yet modestly, successful in helping clients obtain and maintain jobs (Bond, 1992). Successful vocational placement has occurred through Job Clubs and transitional and supported employment programs when clients have had access to continual intervention from mental health professionals convenient to their workplaces (Jacobs and others, 1984; Bond and Dincin, 1986).

Within the past five years, supported employment has grown as a vocational rehabilitation intervention for people with psychiatric disabilities (Anthony and Blanch, 1987). This intervention uses a "place-then-train" rather than a "train-then-place" modality for job placement (*Federal Register*, 1987). Rather than spending lengthy time periods in preparatory, prevocational settings, participants are matched with existing jobs in the real-life community marketplace and are provided with instruction and support to sustain productive participation in the work site. In contrast to the supported employment programs for people with mental retardation, the programs tailored for people with psychiatric disabilities must defer to the client for job decisions and permit the client to obtain supervision and assistance from the rehabilitation practitioner away from the job site. Moreover, persons with psychiatric disabilities often need little on-site training to perform job tasks; instead, these clients tend to need assistance in applying social skills to master the challenges of the work culture and its interpersonal demands (MacDonald-Wilson, Mancuso, Danley, and Anthony, 1989).

The Employment Support Services program at the Boston University Center for Psychiatric Rehabilitation is a supported employment program based on the *choose-get-keep* approach. This approach focuses practitioner efforts on developing and enhancing participants' skills, support, and employment experiences. Derived from tested psychiatric rehabilitation principles, the approach incorporates needed modifications in prevailing supported employment program models (Danley and Anthony, 1987). The Employment Support Services program and its empirical evaluation are described in this chapter.

Program Description

The Employment Support Services program is designed to provide instruction, opportunity, and support for adults eighteen to fifty-five years of age who have a psychiatric diagnosis of a severe mental illness (schizophrenia, manic depression, or other major psychiatric disorder) and whose lives have been seriously disrupted through hospitalizations due to ongoing and recurrent episodes of mental illness. It is the mission of this program to help people with psychiatric disabilities become satisfied and successful in work environments of their choice with the least possible professional support (MacDonald-Wilson, Mancuso, Danley, and Anthony, 1989). The program is staffed by program specialists who have master's degrees in rehabilitation counseling with a specialty in psychiatric rehabilitation. Each specialist provides twenty-four direct service hours per week with an average caseload of fourteen participants.

The Employment Support Services program implements the choose-get-keep approach. This approach is derived from the principles and practices of psychiatric rehabilitation developed by Anthony and others (1990) at Boston University. Their approach to rehabilitation emphasizes person-centered goals; a client-environment match; prescriptive assessment, planning, and intervention; and the development of the unique set of skills and personal supports that an individual needs to be satisfied and successful in selected community settings.

Essentially, the three sets of program activities—choosing, getting, and keeping—parallel the supported employment components described, respectively, as job matching, placement, and training/follow-along (Moon, Grodall, Baccus, and Brooke, 1986). However, the terms choose, get, and keep were selected to focus on participant process rather than on practitioner activity. The goal of choosing is the selection of a job compatible with the participant's values and qualifications. The goal of getting is the acquisition of a job from an employer in a desired competitive work setting. The goal of keeping is the maintenance of employee success and satisfaction through development and enhancement of participant skills and supports.

Inherent to this approach is the principle of mutual responsibility for outcome. Throughout all program activities, the client and the practitioner negotiate to determine various levels of responsibility for selecting, securing, and sustaining employment. These determinations are based on an exploration of the participant's competencies, resources, and preferences, as well as the characteristics of the natural work environment. Similar to the place-train approach, necessary skills and supports are developed or refined in relation to the specific demands of the environment in which the person is working. As discussed by Nisbet and Hagner (1988), the concept of support is defined broadly and includes support provided by job coaches, co-workers, supervisors, attendants, family, and case managers.

Choosing Activities. The three major choosing activities are employment goal setting, job development, and decision making. These activities occur prior to placement but overlap considerably. In fact, some may occur simultaneously. A participant may also recycle through choosing activities once he or she has reached the getting or the keeping phase.

The first choosing activity, setting an employment goal, results in the formulation of a "statement of employment intent," which specifies the client's preferred work activity, work setting, amount of time per week, and target date for employment. For example, a client might state, "I want to work as a library assistant in a small art or music library for twenty-five hours per week by two months from now." To arrive at this goal, the practitioner and participant carefully examine current personal circumstances and relevant or recent work experience. From this investigation, they define the client's values, interests, competencies, and credentials. These are used to define the ingredients of the employment goal. The employment goal anchors the program efforts and focuses the job development process. Although this goal may change over time, it is extremely useful as a mutually determined starting point.

The information gathered is also used to develop a list of personal criteria and general work qualifications. The initial emphasis is on examination of values so that personal criteria can be established for estimating potential job satisfaction. Extreme care is taken to objectify personal criteria so that they are observable and measurable. This process results in a scaled listing of defined personal criteria that is used to evaluate job options in terms of "favorability" (Pierce, Cohen, Anthony, and Cohen, 1980); for instance, favorability may be operationalized by the percentage of time per day on the job that involves work for which there is no prescribed daily routine.

These criteria are used to develop and reflect the unique expectations of the participant. This specificity helps to eliminate ambiguity and confusion. For example, the value "people contact" may have unique meanings for different people. For one person it may be defined as "the percentage of time per day that I do job tasks with co-workers." For another it may mean, "the number of times per day that I speak socially with co-workers."

Although program services may be marketed to employers independently of an individual participant, only those specific jobs are developed that match program participants' unique preferences and qualifications. Ideally, more than one job opportunity is developed for a participant, promoting choice and the possibility of a closer match with his or her ideal employment goal. Once one or more job options are identified, the participant is helped in examining each option, using personal criteria and current qualifications to decide whether the option is a match worthy of further pursuit.

The task of gauging the support of significant others (family members, professionals, friends) for the employment goal is also an essential part of the decision-making process. It is important to note that significant others are engaged in decision making *after* the participant has clarified his or her own goal. This sequence helps to ensure that, while other opinions are considered, the choice is made by the participant. The purpose of gauging support is to identify and project the likelihood of future facilitators and barriers to goal achievement.

Because choosing activities emphasize intense involvement of the participant in the selection of a job and because the process of choice is often difficult for people with psychiatric disability, job matching frequently requires more time than is generally allotted in the prevailing supported employment approaches. Also contributing to the need for increased time are the vocational variability of the population and the difficult, essential task of developing a trusting relationship between the participant and the practitioner. This alliance serves as the basis for all future program efforts (McCrory, 1991). Current data indicate that the time needed for choosing activities ranges from three weeks to six months (MacDonald-Wilson, Mancuso, Danley, and Anthony, 1989).

Getting Activities. Getting activities include placement planning, direct placement, and placement support. Placement planning involves negotiation of responsibility and scheduling times for completion of each of the tasks required to secure a job offer. Placement research has identified placement planning as the single most important factor in obtaining a job for a rehabilitation client (Zadny, 1977).

Based on the placement plan, the practitioner initiates either direct placement activities or placement support. Direct placement tasks require that the practitioner serve as the participant's agent or representative, that is, the practitioner acts on the participant's behalf with potential employer(s). This approach may be used with participants who have good work potential but present themselves poorly in interviewing situations. Placement support tasks help the participant to be his or her own representative with potential employers; for example, the practitioner may teach job-seeking skills to the participant so that he or she can independently obtain the job.

Generally, a combination of direct placement and placement support activities is necessary, depending on the client's interest and skill in independently performing placement tasks, the urgency for securing a job, and the availability of the needed resources. For example, if time allows and the participant's interest is high, instead of using the strategies needed to market a program participant directly with the employer, the practitioner can teach the program participant to apply and use these skills in presenting his or her strengths to the employer in person.

It has been our experience that disability disclosure is frequently a major concern for people with psychiatric disabilities and may require much discussion. If the disability is disclosed prior to hiring, either the client must be taught how to describe the impact of the disability positively, or the practitioner must be able to educate the employer and overcome any employer objections. Because psychiatric impairment may be invisible and because stigma against people with psychiatric histories continues to be widespread, many people with psychiatric disability may elect *not* to disclose the fact that they have a disability to prospective employers.

Keeping Activities. To help participants keep their jobs, interventions are needed to build interpersonal skills demanded by the social dimensions of a particular work environment. Keeping activities of supported employment include skill development, service coordination, and employer consultation. To develop participant skills, practitioners use either direct skills teaching or skills programming. When the program participant must acquire a new skill, the practitioner develops and delivers a well-planned lesson, created specifically for the program participant. Skills programming is selected when the participant can already perform a particular skill but has difficulty using the skill as often or as well as needed in the work situation (Cohen, Danley, and Nemec, 1985). These skill development interventions have been described comprehensively by Anthony, Farkas, and Cohen (1990).

Service coordination, another keeping intervention option, involves the tasks of arranging for and facilitating the use of resources exterior to the work site that the program participant needs for success and satisfaction on the job. Service coordination activities consist of accompanying the participant for crisis intervention, medication management, or other psychiatric services, as well as linking the participant to existing social, housing, and financial resources or creating new resources (Cohen, Vitalo, Anthony, and Pierce, 1980).

The third type of keeping intervention is employer consultation. This intervention includes activities that help employers make adjustments in the job or work setting in order to accommodate the participant's disability and increase productivity. Such accommodations are required by Section

504C of the Rehabilitation Act of 1986. However, employers and supervisors commonly lack the skills and knowledge required to make reasonable changes that facilitate employee functioning. Through consultation with the employer, the practitioner who knows the client's strengths and limitations can make creative, inexpensive suggestions that are mutually beneficial (MacDonald-Wilson, Mancuso, Danley, and Anthony, 1989). Reasonable accommodations of the workplace for people with psychiatric disabilities are relatively simple and low cost, such as granting time off for psychiatrist appointments or access to the telephone for crisis consultation and counseling calls (Mancuso, 1990). Skill development, service coordination, and employer consultation may all be needed simultaneously when problem situations emerge on the job.

Efficacy of the Choose-Get-Keep Approach

In a recent study, of nineteen participants with psychiatric disabilities who received the choose-get-keep intervention over a one-year period, seven (or 37 percent) of the participants had schizophrenia, ten (or 53 percent) had manic depression, and two (or 10 percent) had other major psychiatric disorders. Of the nineteen participants, seventeen (or 90 percent) were employed at least once, fourteen (or 74 percent) were consecutively employed for a minimum of sixty days during the one year of the project, and eight (or 42 percent) were employed at the end of one year. Of the eleven who were not working after one year, seven were attending or pursuing further education or training. These results and client population were similar to those reported by Bond (1992) in which 80 percent of the clients receiving supported employment services were employed at least once, and 52 percent were employed at the end of the one-year period.

The number of participants employed and their hours worked increased dramatically over the first three quarters of participation and decreased slightly in the fourth quarter and at end point. It is noteworthy that of those who left jobs, only one left due to unsatisfactory job performance. A repeated-measures analysis of variance, with time as the repeated measure, was performed on employment status and hours worked per week. Both employment status ($F[5,90] = 6.29$, $p = .0001$) and hours worked ($F[5,75] = 5.41$, $p = .0001$) showed a significant positive linear trend over time. Earnings also increased from a mean of \$2,286 in the year prior to enrollment to \$3,069 in the year after enrollment, but this increase was not statistically significant. Most participants who were working held semiskilled or clerical positions and this characteristic did not change over time. Examples of job titles held include medical records librarian, clerk typist, research assistant, maintenance person, and personal care attendant. An examination of clinical and social status revealed no significant change within the one-year time period.

Neither demographic characteristics of the clients nor diagnosis predicted employment status at quarters three and four and at end point, using regression models. Controlling for all other variables in the model, only age significantly predicted employment status at quarter four ($t[1]$ = 2.19, p = .04). Younger subjects more often became employed. Controlling for all other variables in the model, we found that the factor of whether or not subjects required help with basic living skills significantly predicted employment status at quarters three ($t[1]$ = 2.46, p = .03) and four ($t[1]$ = 2.2, p = .04). The difference was in the expected direction, with those not needing help with residential adjustment more often employed. However, as found in other studies (Jacobs, Collier, and Wissusik, this volume; Bond, 1992), the best predictor of employment status was employment history.

Costs for psychiatric treatment services to the nineteen clients in this project decreased by 47 percent, while costs for community support and rehabilitation services, excluding the direct supported employment program costs, decreased by 24 percent. However, while utilization of clinical services decreased by 44 percent, utilization of other forms of community services increased by 53 percent, due largely to advocacy by program staff.

When the costs of $7,128 per participant for program operation were included, total costs for community services increased slightly. Although participants experienced an average reduction of $933 in public benefits in one year, this and other reductions in service costs did not fully offset cost increases for the program. Future program evaluation will determine whether cost-efficiency improves as caseload size increases and clients stabilize in employment.

Case Example: William

William is a Caucasian male, thirty-nine years of age, with a diagnosis of chronic, paranoid schizophrenia. Upon entering the program, he was taking three psychotropic medications and reported mild to moderate symptom interference. When he entered the program, William lived at home with his parents. He was working as a volunteer janitor for a local psychosocial program.

Between 1974 and 1978, William was hospitalized twice, each time for a period of twenty weeks. His last hospitalization was approximately two and one-half years before project enrollment. Since that time, he has continued outpatient therapy and has a state-funded case manager. He had used emergency services twice during the year prior to program enrollment.

During the five-year period prior to entering the program, William reported that he had held nine jobs. Each of these jobs ended when he resigned due to dissatisfaction or increased symptomatology. Job tenure ranged from two to ten months. William's initial reason for wanting to enter the program was to get a job that he could keep for longer than ten months.

Choosing. William and his program specialist initially explored his employment history to determine his personal criteria and qualifications. William identified three personal criteria: (1) working with money, (2) working where there were lots of people, and (3) working indoors. When examining options, William identified cashiering as a preferred work activity. His first stated employment goal was "I want to work as a cashier in an indoor business that serves many people for twenty hours per week within three months."

The job developer, using William's criteria and qualifications as a guide, identified a cashier job on the Boston University campus. William investigated this job, found it to be a good fit to the personal definitions of his criteria, and decided to pursue employment.

Getting. Initially, the job was developed by the program specialist. However, both William and the employer wanted a hiring interview. William was coached on how to present himself affirmatively and received a job offer subsequent to the interview. Since William's employer knew of his participation in our service program, disability disclosure was made.

Keeping. Once the job choice was clear, skill and support needs were identified. A functional assessment identified the need for wake-up calls to help William surmount the morning lethargy caused by his illness and medications. It was also found that William needed instruction regarding appropriate dress for the work site and management of his newly earned wages. It was also necessary to negotiate a reasonable accommodation for William. Because his medications left his mouth dry, a request was made and granted that William be permitted to drink liquids while working. This violated the regulations of the cafeteria, but the regulation was waived as an accommodation.

William remained in this position successfully for two months. Then, due to a cutback in staffing, and through no fault of his own, his employment was terminated. As a result, William reinstituted his choosing activities, this time assuming a more active role as his own job developer. Personal criteria in hand, he investigated several jobs and decided to become an independent newspaper agent, selling two major city newspapers at an indoor subway station. Currently, he works twenty-four hours per week and has done so for over one year.

When he had worked for twelve months, two months beyond his previous "record," William invited the program staff who had provided support to a celebration lunch. He has remained out of the hospital and has had no further contact with crisis services. He has also moved into a subsidized apartment near his parents' home.

William continues to receive employment support and consultation, off-site, to ensure his job success. Primarily, he needs telephone support, evenings and weekends, to help him redirect feelings and thoughts that might interfere with his work. He also continues to require assistance with money management issues. Until recently, William's public benefit status with the Social Security Administration had remained unchanged. However, due to his increased income and steady employment pattern, these benefits are now in jeopardy. The program specialist is helping William utilize Social Security work incentives such as development of a Plan for Achieving Self-Support.

Summary

Increasing numbers of people with psychiatric disabilities are residing in communities rather than in inpatient settings. They are also becoming more aware of the benefits of working and of their legal right to employment with accommodations. Traditional work preparation programs have failed to result in employment for many people with psychiatric disabilities. However, supported employment, when modified to reflect the basic principles and practices of effective psychiatric rehabilitation, has been shown to result in employment benefits for participants at a reasonable cost to providers. With supported employment methodologies such as the choose-get-keep approach, providers can do much to help people with psychiatric disabilities reap the many social and financial benefits of employment and achieve their community living goals.

References

Anthony, W. A., and Blanch, A. K. "Supported Employment for Persons Who Are Psychiatrically Disabled: A Historical and Conceptual Perspective." *Psychosocial Rehabilitation Journal,* 1987, *11* (2), 5–23.

Anthony, W. A., Cohen, M. R., and Danley, K. S. "The Psychiatric Rehabilitation Approach as Applied to Vocational Rehabilitation." In J. A. Ciardiello and M. D. Bell (eds.), *Vocational Rehabilitation of Persons with Prolonged Psychiatric Disorders.* Baltimore, Md.: Johns Hopkins University Press, 1988.

Anthony, W. A., Farkas, M. D., and Cohen, M. R. *Psychiatric Rehabilitation.* Boston: Boston University, Center for Psychiatric Rehabilitation, 1990.

Bond, G. R. "Vocational Rehabilitation." In R. P. Liberman (ed.), *Handbook of Psychiatric Rehabilitation.* Elmsford, N.Y.: Pergamon, 1992.

Bond, G. R., and Dincin, J. "Accelerating Entry into Transitional Employment in a Psychosocial Rehabilitation Agency." *Rehabilitation Psychiatry,* 1986, *31,* 143–154.

Cohen, M. R., Danley, K. S., and Nemec, P. B. *Directory of Technical Assistance Resources for Community Support Systems.* Boston: Center for Psychiatric Rehabilitation, Boston University, 1985.

Cohen, M. R., Vitalo, R. L., Anthony, W. A., and Pierce, R. M. *The Skills of Community Service Coordination.* Psychiatric Rehabilitation Practice Series, vol. 6. Baltimore, Md.: University Park Press, 1980.

Danley, K. S. *Supported Employment Research Project.* Final report. Boston: Center for Psychiatric Rehabilitation, Boston University, 1991.

Danley, K. S., and Anthony, W. A. "The Choose-Get-Keep Model: Serving Severely Psychiatrically Disabled People." *American Rehabilitation,* 1987, *13* (4), 6–9, 27–29.

Dion, G. L., and Anthony, W. A. "Research in Psychiatric Rehabilitation: A Review of Exper-imental and Quasi-Experimental Studies." *Rehabilitation Counseling Bulletin,* 1987, *30,* 177–203.

Federal Register. "The State-Supported Employment Services Program." Aug. 14, 1987, no. 30546.

Jacobs, H. E., Collier, R., and Wissusik, D. "The Job Finding Module." In R. P. Liberman (ed.), *Handbook of Psychiatric Rehabilitation.* Elmsford, N.Y.: Pergamon, 1992.

Jacobs, H. E., Kardashian, S., Kreinbring, R. K., Ponder, R., and Simpson, A. R. "A Skills-Oriented Model for Facilitating Employment Among Psychiatrically Disabled Persons." *Rehabilitation Counseling Bulletin,* 1984, *28,* 87–96.

McCrory, D. "The Rehabilitation Alliance." *Journal of Vocational Rehabilitation,* 1991, *1* (3), 58–66.

MacDonald-Wilson, K. L., Mancuso, L. L., Danley, K. S., and Anthony, W. A. "Supported Employment for People with Psychiatric Disability." *Journal of Applied Rehabilitation Coun-seling,* 1989, *20* (3), 50–57.

Mancuso, L. "Reasonable Accommodation for People with Psychiatric Disability." *Psychosocial Rehabilitation Journal,* 1990, *14* (2), 3–19.

Moon, S., Grodall, P., Baccus, M., and Brooke, V. *The Supported Work Model of Competitive Employment for Citizens with Severe Handicaps.* Richmond: Rehabilitation Research and Training Center, Virginia Commonwealth University, 1986.

Nisbet, J., and Hagner, J. "Natural Supports in the Workplace: A Reexamination of Supported Employment." *Journal of the Association for Persons with Severe Handicaps,* 1988, *13* (4), 260–267.

Pierce, R. M., Cohen, M. R., Anthony, W. A., Cohen, B. F., and Friel, T. W. *The Skills of Career Counseling.* Psychiatric Rehabilitation Practice Series, vol. 4. Baltimore, Md.: University Park Press, 1980.

Rogers, E. S., Walsh, D., Danley, K. S., and Smith, K. *Massachusetts Client Preference Assessment.* Final report. Boston: Center for Psychiatric Rehabilitation, Boston University, 1991.

Unger, K. V., and Anthony, W. A. "Are Families Satisfied with Services to Young Adult Chronic Patients? A Recent Survey and a Proposed Alternative." In B. Pepper and H. Ryglewicz (eds.), *Advances in Treating the Young Adult Chronic Patient.* New Directions for Mental Health Services, no. 21. San Francisco: Jossey-Bass, 1984.

Zadny, J. J. "A Review of Research on Job Placement." *Rehabilitation Counseling Bulletin,* 1977, *21,* 150–158.

KAREN S. DANLEY, *Ph.D., is director of Career Achievement Services at the Center for Psychiatric Rehabilitation, Boston University, Brookline, Massachu-setts, and principal investigator for the Supported Employment Research Project.*

KEN SCIARAPPA, *M.S., is research associate at the Center for Psychiatric Rehabil-itation where he conducted all of the data analysis and cost-benefit methodology cited in this chapter.*

KIM MACDONALD-WILSON, *M.A., is director of Career Support Services, including supported employment, and functions as assistant project director for the Sup-ported Employment Research Project at the Center for Psychiatric Rehabilitation.*

While institution-bound programs in horticulture therapy were appropriate for the era in which long-term hospitalization was the primary mode of psychiatric treatment, the supported employment paradigm updates this mode of treatment for the current era of community psychiatry.

The Growth of Supported Employment from Horticulture Therapy in the Veterans' Garden

Jerome V. Vaccaro, Ida Cousino, Robert Vatcher

A renaissance in vocational rehabilitation is marked by the emergence of the supported employment movement. The supported employment initiative stems from the understanding that individuals with psychiatric disabilities require ongoing services, such as training in the skills necessary to maintain employment, once they secure competitive employment. It deemphasizes the importance of prevocational training, advocating instead a "place-then-train" approach. Patients are placed in employment settings and then offered training and other necessary mental health support services necessary to maintain their positions. In its fully applied form, individuals are offered services indefinitely, with job coaches visiting them at their workplaces to help them learn and retain the skills that they need to sustain employment. The following case vignette illustrates the type of mental health and rehabilitation services that are helpful to these individuals:

> Jim, a forty-one-year-old veteran of the Vietnam War, had been unable to obtain and then keep a job since he was discharged from the military. His military tenure was marked by exemplary service, with a duty assignment

The authors acknowledge the efforts of the following individuals: Don Flinn, M.D., and William Anderson for their administrative support, Mary Sue Milliken and Susan Feniger of City Restaurant for helping us develop our product lines and for their consistent community support, and the Veterans' Affairs Medical Center Voluntary Service for their ongoing support of our activities.

that required him to process the remains of troops killed in Vietnam. As a result of this experience, he was left with symptoms of post-traumatic stress disorder (PTSD). He reported recurring nightmares, almost constant anxiety, irritability, mood swings, and social isolation. He entered the Veterans' Garden program during one of his frequent hospitalizations for suicidal threats and depression. Before entering the program, he had been hospitalized an average of three times per year for about a decade.

Jim was a very responsible worker in the garden, but a number of deficits were noted in the areas of social interactions, especially with his superiors, distractibility, and work stamina in that he could not sustain a task for very long or complete tasks on time. This slowness in accomplishing his tasks frustrated him greatly and contributed to his poor self-esteem. He noted that this frustration would often lead him to "mouth off," as he put it, to his superiors. Once his work stamina improved, he was hired to work on the gardening crew of a local university. Before he started the job, Jim asked that his new boss meet his job coach, Vince. Vince helped Jim speak with his superior about his strengths and weaknesses, specifically outlining his troubles with authority. Over the next several weeks, Vince made regular visits to Jim on the job, assisting him by teaching him a structured problem-solving technique to solve difficult work challenges. Once a week, Jim came to a skills-training class run by Vince for patients in the Veterans' Garden and the supported employment program. In this group, patients discussed their experiences at work and, through the use of role play and the structured problem-solving process, developed new coping strategies. For example, Jim was able to work out plans to negotiate his work assignments, advocate for recognition from his supervisor for well-done tasks, and develop coping strategies to deal with experiences that triggered his PTSD symptoms.

The Veterans' Garden, developed ten years ago within the Rehabilitation Medicine Service of the West Los Angeles Veterans Affairs (VA) Medical Center, Brentwood (Psychiatric) Division, provides seriously mentally ill individuals with prevocational and vocational training, work hardening, and supported and transitional employment in a horticultural setting. The garden is predicated on the importance of evaluating and meeting the needs of mentally disabled individuals by weaving services into a comprehensive, continuous fabric and encouraging informed self-determination among users of the services (Vaccaro, Pitts, and Wallace, 1991; Danley, Rogers, and Novas, 1989).

Most participants are outpatients and carry multiple psychiatric diagnoses, including schizophrenia, personality disorders, PTSD, and drug dependence. The program is located on the hospital grounds, with a fifteen-acre vegetable farm, a greenhouse, a lathe house, and a small classroom for didactic instruction. The farm grows vegetables, herbs, flowers, and ornamental plants for sale. Sales activities are varied and include contracts for produce supply to several local gourmet restaurants, sales at farmers' markets, and a service in which we sell floral arrangements to staff of the medical center. Guided by the multidimensional model for psychiatric rehabilitation articulated by Anthony and Liberman (1991), we help individuals remediate their disabilities through the provision of skills training and environmental support. The major components of our program include training in social and independent living skills, horticultural skills training, work hardening experiences, transitional employment, and job support and coaching. Participants ready for competitive employment have access to a Job Club (Jacobs, Collier, and Wissusik, this volume) in which training and support in job search and interviewing skills are provided.

For several years, the program was entirely based on the grounds of the VA Medical Center, offering therapeutic activities designed to give patients sheltered work experiences. When the current chief assumed her role, attention was shifted to include more activities that simulate the competitive employment environment: an expanded range of products, including herbs and vegetables, house and landscape plants, and flowers; opportunities to sell produce to restaurants and the general public; and a service that delivers floral arrangements throughout the medical center. Over the past year, supported employment activities have been initiated, a psychiatrist has led a skills-training group designed to teach members the skills that they need to successfully maintain their jobs, counselors have engaged in job development and job coaching, and we have increased our community visibility through public sales and employer consultation.

Horticulture Therapy and the Veterans' Garden

The horticultural rehabilitation program of the Veterans' Garden is divided into five interlocking components: work skills and stamina assessment, work skills training, social skills training for the work environment, didactic horticultural training, and job support and coaching.

Work Skills and Stamina Assessment. In this phase, lasting from several days to two weeks, individuals are evaluated by staff and other patients for initiation and maintenance of work tasks, social and independent living skills, and aptitude for and interest in horticultural work. They are observed working in the fields and greenhouses, at plant and vegetable sales, and in skills-training classes. They are also engaged in a goal-setting process in which they identify their future vocational aspirations. At the end of the assessment, they are given clear, concise feedback about their performance, and a plan is developed for their continued involvement in the program. The plan includes activities such as learning work-specific and social and independent living skills, horticultural terms and techniques, and time management.

Work Skills Training. During this phase, individuals are coached about appropriate work behaviors such as arriving for work on time, planning and performing work tasks according to a schedule, and getting along with superiors, subordinates, and peers. One of the program participants is assigned a supervisory position and oversees others in their work. This individual is one of the patients in the program, typically someone who is at an advanced worker level. The supervisor schedules work activities, plans sales, arranges for visitor tours, and assigns participants to their work routines.

Social Skills for the Workplace. We hold a regular social skills training group at the work site, modeled after the Successful Living format articulated by Hierholzer and Liberman (1986). We use behavioral and learning techniques to teach participants the skills that they need to interact effectively in the workplace. Participants identify their interpersonal problems or situations that they would like to improve, and group members use role play and structured problem-solving techniques to redress these problems. The following case vignette illustrates this process:

> Bill is a forty-two-year-old man diagnosed as suffering from schizophrenia and PTSD. He has been in treatment for much of the past twenty years since leaving the military. His psychotic symptoms have been under control since he was stabilized on a low-dose regimen of antipsychotic medication. He is currently being treated by a special team for his PTSD.
>
> Bill has held a number of jobs but has never been able to maintain employment for longer than several months at a time. His usual pattern is to secure employment, perform well on the job, but then lose the job after an explosive episode with a co-worker. This pattern repeated itself at the Veterans' Garden, and he recently had several arguments with his peers.
>
> In a group skills-training session, Bill said that he would like to "fix this temper of mine." He related an incident that had occurred earlier that day, in which he had screamed at a co-worker when this worker did not give him a tool that he needed. He and his co-worker had been having difficulty getting along for several weeks, and this incident seemed to be the culmination of these problems.
>
> The psychiatrist leading the social skills group helped Bill clarify the problems leading up to the outburst. Bill said, "This guy's been trying to get my goat and have me explode since I got my promotion and he had to start listening to me." Bill had been anxious about his new supervisory responsibilities and felt uncomfortable about his ability to get along with his peers and superiors. During the group sessions, he identified alternative responses to becoming irritated and yelling at his co-worker, including asking his supervisor for help in assigning tasks, speak-

ing directly with his co-worker about problems before they get out of hand, and asking workers at his own supervisory level about how they handle similar problems. Bill then developed a plan to implement each of these activities, and the group leader engaged him in role-play exercises to practice these exchanges. In the next session, Bill reported to the group that he had successfully negotiated the difficulties with his co-worker, and that he now felt better about himself and his new position.

Didactic Component. Classes are held each week so that participants gain the knowledge necessary to work in the horticultural and landscaping trade. The classes are held on-site and cover such issues as plant identification and characteristics, irrigation systems, and landscape planning. We also hold reading and English classes. In addition, participants are familiarized with and referred to off-site classes at community colleges and other schools.

Job Support and Coaching. The new addition to our program is the capacity to assist participants, once they secure employment, in maintaining employment. We view this as an essential element in the rehabilitation process, even though resource constraints delayed its development and implementation. It began with the establishment of a working agreement with the University of California, Los Angeles (UCLA), to have several of our program participants work in a UCLA landscaping unit. The placement begins with a short training phase in which participants are educated about the specific requirements and unique demands of the job. As described by Danley, Sciarappa, and MacDonald-Wilson (this volume), we employ three types of interventions in the job-coaching phase: skill development, as denoted in the description of the group intervention above; service coordination, a type of clinical case management similar to that described in other of our programs (Vaccaro, Liberman, Wallace, and Blackwell, this volume), the goal of which is to ensure that appropriate clinical and educational services are provided to maximize learning and minimize relapse; and employer consultation.

During the ongoing phases of employment, participants are visited by a job coach, who guides the worker in the use of the work and social and independent living skills that he or she learned in the Veterans' Garden. It is our hope that this effort will improve job maintenance of program participants who are placed in competitive employment. The support is provided indefinitely and also includes attendance at regular alumni meetings, modeled after the social skills training for the workplace group described above. The following case vignette illustrates this process:

> Hal, a forty-year-old man, was diagnosed as having bipolar affective disorder. Relapses are characterized by increasing irritability that pro-

gresses to euphoria, paranoid ideation that progresses to delusional states, disorganized thinking, impulsive behavior such as spending large sums of money, auditory hallucinations, and pressured speech. His symptoms have been refractory to standard treatment, necessitating long trials of novel psychopharmacological agents combined with psychosocial interventions designed so that he is able to seek treatment at the first sign of relapse. Since undergoing this treatment combination, he has experienced only one full relapse in the past year, compared to an average of four in each of the preceding five years.

In the past, these symptomatic impairments have led to abrupt termination from employment. Hal became so demoralized as a result of this cycle of good interepisode functioning, during which time he was able to secure employment, disrupted by periods of severe symptomatic impairment, that he gave up looking for work. After attending several sessions of the social skills for the workplace group, the psychiatrist who led the group and his vocational counselor suggested that he enter the new supported employment program. He agreed, and although very skeptical about his own prognosis, performed quite well on the job. His supervisors said that he was one of their most productive workers. Initially, a problem developed when his fears that he would fail led him to refuse several job assignments. His vocational counselor met with him and his supervisor and established a trial period, during which time Hal would attempt one of these job assignments and receive frequent visits from the counselor for support and guidance. Once he successfully accomplished these tasks, he accepted greater responsibility and eventually was assigned to manicure the gardens of the chancellor, a prestigious but difficult assignment. Hal and his supervisor established an "inside joke" about his pattern of first refusing and then accepting and performing well at tasks.

Summary and Future Directions

The Veterans' Garden is a vocational rehabilitation program combining work skills training, work hardening, social and independent living skills training, and supported employment. Designed for individuals with serious mental illnesses, the program is guided by a multidimensional model of mental illness in which we assume that individuals can be taught coping skills and can benefit from environmental supports that buffer the adverse effects of vulnerability and stressors.

We have found that the use of a horticultural setting enhances outcomes in a number of ways. The negative symptoms of illnesses such as amotivation and social isolation are overcome through patients' involvement in a wide range of activities and through use of reinforcers such as payment for their work, public recognition of their sales work, and increased responsibility. Many individuals with serious mental illnesses are in poor physical condition. Horticultural work enhances their motor skills and builds physical strength. The cognitive disabilities of their illnesses, such as poor attention, concentration, cognitive processing, and planning skills, are also targeted for intervention in a systematic manner.

Our program is in its early stages. Research on the effectiveness of our interventions will look at a number of areas: successful placement in competitive employment, decreased relapses and hospital recidivism, increased quality of life, and greater success in meeting individualized vocational goals. We plan to carefully study the new supported employment element of our program, articulating a model that incorporates social skills training and case management activities with accepted supported employment interventions.

References

Anthony, W. A., and Liberman, R. P. "Principles and Practice of Psychiatric Rehabilitation." In R. P. Liberman (ed.), *Handbook of Psychiatric Rehabilitation*. Elmsford, N.Y.: Pergamon, 1991.

Bond, G. R. "Vocational Rehabilitation for Persons with Severe Mental Illness: Past, Present, and Future." In R. P. Liberman (ed.), *Handbook of Psychiatric Rehabilitation*. Elmsford, N.Y.: Pergamon, 1991.

Danley, K. S., Rogers, E. S., and Novas, D. B. "A Psychiatric Rehabilitation Approach to Vocational Rehabilitation." In M. D. Farkas and W. A. Anthony (eds.), *Psychiatric Rehabilitation Programs: Putting Theory into Practice*. Baltimore, Md.: Johns Hopkins University Press, 1989.

Hierholzer, R. W., and Liberman, R. P. "Successful Living: A Social Skills and Problem-Solving Group for the Chronically Mentally Ill." *Hospital and Community Psychiatry*, 1986, *37*, 913–918.

Vaccaro, J. V., Pitts, D. B., and Wallace, C. J. "Functional Assessment." In R. P. Liberman (ed.), *Handbook of Psychiatric Rehabilitation*. Elmsford, N.Y.: Pergamon, 1991.

JEROME V. VACCARO, M.D., is assistant professor of psychiatry at the UCLA School of Medicine, assistant chief of the Rehabilitation Medicine Service of the West Los Angeles VA Medical Center, Brentwood Division, and investigator in the UCLA Clinical Research Center for Schizophrenia and Psychiatric Rehabilitation. He leads a skills-training group at the Veterans' Garden and provides psychiatric consultation and liaison to its patients.

IDA COUSINO, O.T.R., C.H.T., is chief of the Veterans' Garden. She is a certified horticultural therapist and registered occupational therapist whose mental health career grew out of many years of advocacy experience for the United Farm Workers' Union. She designed the programmatic elements of the Veterans' Garden and has successfully generated widespread community support for its activities.

ROBERT VATCHER, C.H.T., is assistant chief of the Veterans' Garden. He is a certified horticultural therapist who ran a successful community nursery before joining the Veterans' Garden.

*Developed from eight years of research, the Job-Finding Module
is designed to help persons with disabilities who are capable of
returning to the work force obtain competitive community
employment.*

The Job-Finding Module: Training Skills for Seeking Competitive Community Employment

Harvey E. Jacobs, Rosemary Collier, Donald Wissusik

The Job-Finding Module is designed to help persons capable of competitive community employment find work. The module emerged from ten years of research and development, as well as from clinical experience in understanding the process of vocational restoration for persons with mental disabilities. The task of getting a job requires a myriad of skills and prerequisite attitudes and preparation. For example, the job seeker must be medically and physically capable of the rigors of work. Psychiatric symptoms must be under control so as to not interfere with work capacity. Prevoca-

The Job-Finding Club research and development project and the Job-Finding Module were supported in part by research grants from the National Institute of Disability and Rehabilitation Research and the Social Security Administration awarded to Robert Paul Liberman, M.D. (principal investigator) and Harvey E. Jacobs, Ph.D. (project director). The authors acknowledge the participation of Susan Kardashian, M.A., C.R.C., Andy Baracco, M.A., C.R.C., Ron Ponder, M.A., C.R.C., Jeff Pass, M.A., David Novak, and Magdeline Fitzpatrick, who have been instrumental in the success of the Clinical Job Finding Club program at the VA Medical Center in West Los Angeles. Project research assistance was provided by Derek Burkeman, B.A., Claudia Dorrington, M.S., Linda Lee, B.A., and Debra Stackman, B.A. We also gratefully acknowledge the assistance of Richard Halmy in the production of the module's training video.

Reprints and information on the Job-Finding Module can be obtained from Harvey E. Jacobs, Ph.D., Drucker Brain Injury Center, Moss Rehabilitation Hospital, 1200 West Tabor Road, Philadelphia, PA 19141.

tional competencies, including a stable place to live, the ability to work with others, punctuality, appropriate personal hygiene, adequate transportation, and stamina, must be available. Work skills must meet community standards, or someone else will be hired. Finally, finding a job and keeping a job are two different sets of skills. The offer of a position is not a promise of job security, only the chance to go to work. A person who cannot perform the technical skills of the job, get along with others, or follow instructions will quickly find out that the first day at work can also be the last.

Accordingly, the Job-Finding Module was designed to be *one* element of an effective vocational rehabilitation system, not to comprise the entire system. People who do not possess adequate personal or vocational skills are, initially, better served by other components of the rehabilitation continuum (Jacobs, 1988; Jacobs, Donahoe, and Falloon, 1985). On the other hand, those who are ready for competitive community employment may find the program highly effective for returning to meaningful work. Before describing the components of the Job-Finding Module, we summarize its origins.

Origins of the Job-Finding Module

The Job Club approach was originally developed by Azrin, Flores, and Kaplan (1975) as an alternative to traditional job-seeking programs. Azrin and his colleagues noted the inefficiency of most job placement services, where one counselor is assigned the task of finding jobs for many people. First, this arrangement creates a dependent role for clients who wait for someone else to locate jobs. Second, it places the job-seeking burden on a vocational counselor who is already busy (and employed)! Azrin and his colleagues sought to develop a program that would support and motivate unemployed persons. After all, these people have the most time available to look for a job and would most directly benefit from their own efforts.

Understanding the difficulties in conducting a concerted job search, Azrin and his colleagues designed the Job Club as a supportive environment. The program provided clients with an office setting conducive for a job search, supplies, fresh job leads, and structured contact with vocational counselors. In return, clients were expected to devote full-time effort to their job searches. The admonition "finding a job is a full time job" was highlighted at the first orientation session of the Job Club. Preliminary results from the program were very favorable, with upward of 85 percent successful job placement for persons without disabilities. Subsequent reports from Azrin and his colleagues have documented the continued clinical and economic efficacy of the program among nondisabled and mixed normal-disabled populations (Azrin, 1978; Azrin, Kaplan, and Flores, 1975; Azrin and Phillip, 1979; Azrin and Besalel, 1980).

The Brentwood Job-Finding Club

The preliminary Job Club findings offered promise for persons with difficult employment challenges, and in 1981, the Brentwood VA Hospital Job-Finding Club was modified to meet the specific needs of persons with psychiatric disabilities. Similar to the "generic" Job Club model, the Brentwood Job-Finding Club presented a structured environment to help individuals find their own competitive community employment. The program operated five days per week, and participants were required to attend daily, until they secured employment or dropped out of the program. The resources required to find a job were provided by the program, but each person took responsibility for his or her own job search.

Critical components of the program were also revised to meet the specific cognitive, emotional, symptomatic, and social support needs of persons with psychiatric disabilities. Hence, job-seeking skills training, the first phase of the program, utilized competency-based training procedures in small group sessions to maximize attention. Socially validated materials were also used to make training more realistic. Most important, participants were given easy access to members of psychiatric treatment teams, including vocational rehabilitation counselors who had extensive experience serving the mentally ill.

Following job-seeking skills training, participants began looking for jobs on a daily basis. The project provided a workplace conducive to the job search, fresh job leads, frequent contact with vocational counselors, daily goal-setting and problem-solving sessions, and a monetary incentive system to encourage consistent participation. Early experience in the Brentwood Job Finding Club indicated that clients required individualized assistance in setting daily goals, solving novel problems, maintaining motivation, establishing personal networks of job lead contacts in light of their diminished social contacts, and learning how to use available vocational resources. Program modifications were made to address each of these challenges, as well as needs for social and independent living skills such as personal finances, living arrangements, and interpersonal communication.

Job-Finding Club Outcomes

Preliminary results of the Brentwood Job Club among military veterans with psychiatric disabilities showed that 65 percent of all participants secured either competitive community employment or job-related training in an average of twenty-seven days (Jacobs and others, 1984). This figure contrasts with the 5 to 15 percent job placement rate noted for persons leaving most inpatient psychiatric treatment settings (Anthony, Buell, Sharratt, and Althoff, 1972; Anthony, Cohen, and Vitalo, 1978; Anthony and

Jansen, 1984). Later outcome studies of the Brentwood Job Club with a broader array of persons with psychiatric disabilities from both institutional and community settings have noted placement rates between 35 and 60 percent (Mitchell, Jacobs, and Yen, 1987; Jacobs and others, 1991). The cost per placement in the Job Club has ranged from $400 to $600 according to the economic models used. These costs are about five times less than the costs ascribed to more traditional, individual counselor-client placement models.

Key factors affecting outcome have included job history, job interview skills, diagnosis, type of disability benefits, independent living skills, and job goals. The strongest correlate of program outcome has been vocational history. Persons with stronger work histories generally did better than persons with poorer histories. Job placement rates for persons with psychiatric disorders, such as schizophrenia and bipolar disorder, were approximately one-half to one-third of the rates of persons with substance abuse or depressive disorders. An evaluation of program results among persons receiving either Supplemental Security Income (SSI) or Social Security Disability Insurance (SSDI) noted higher employment rates among the SSDI beneficiaries than among the SSI recipients. However, SSDI beneficiaries also tended to have better job histories than those of individuals receiving SSI. Persons with stable places to live, stronger social support, and reliable transportation also generally did better than those who had to devote greater attention to daily subsistence issues rather than to their job searches. Finally, persons with focused and attainable job goals, based on their skills and experience, were more often successful in seeking employment than were those with vague or unrealistic aspirations.

The Job-Finding Module

Findings from the Brentwood Job-Finding Club resulted in numerous requests for its dissemination to other rehabilitation settings. Over the past two years, a module has been developed to facilitate program adaptation to a variety of different settings. The module consists of four components: (1) a technical manual on the design and operation of Job Finding Clubs, (2) a job-seeking skills training curriculum, (3) a client workbook, and (4) a video training tape that demonstrates selected job-seeking skills. After completing training, clients can enter structured job searches to secure employment.

Job-Finding Club Technical Manual. The technical manual describes how to establish a Job-Finding Club for persons with psychiatric, neurological, or learning disabilities or other impairments who require special training. The manual includes a philosophical overview; instructions on the design, development, and operation of the program; basic forms; and clinical procedures. Using this manual, vocational staff are able to evaluate the applicability of the program to their particular setting, determine which program components can be implemented on-site, identify the start-up and operating costs of the program, estimate client flow and staffing needs, and learn how to operate the overall program.

Job-Seeking Skills Training Curriculum: Trainer's Manual. This manual covers the job-seeking skills training curriculum and includes detailed descriptions of training procedures, materials, assessment protocols, and client exercises. It is also integrated with the training video and the client workbook. The manual is programmed to guide trainers through each of the seven skill areas in the curriculum. Each skill area begins with an introduction that highlights the goals and content of the section. Step-by-step instructions are provided for each task, including how to introduce each section to clients, when to incorporate the videotape into training, question-and-answer sessions, workbook exercises, role plays, and other assignments. Answers to questions, appropriate responses, and remedial exercises are also provided.

Client training is competency based, and socially validated materials are used throughout the module. Training segments are brief and contain concrete examples with frequent feedback to maintain client participation. Special sensitivity is devoted to the needs and problems that persons with disabilities face during the job search.

Skill Areas of the Job-Finding Module

With a group of eight participants, training requires approximately thirty hours over a five-day period. However, the program is flexible enough to be used in one-on-one training situations as well as with larger groups. The seven skill areas include helping clients determine if they are ready to return to work, what types of jobs are best for them, how to identify sources of job leads, how to contact employers, how to fill out job applications, job interviewing, and how to negotiate a job offer. Combined, these skill areas equip clients with the knowledge and skills required to seek competitive community employment. Individual skill areas can be used independently for other vocational situations such as supported employment programs, or to address specific skill deficits in individual clients.

Skill Area 1: "Are You Ready for a Job?" Clients are introduced to the Job Finding Club by the counselor who reviews basic program goals and helps clients determine if they have the requisite abilities and living conditions to find and secure employment. These include lifestyle issues such as housing, transportation, and personal schedules; personal performance issues such as physical and mental health; and an understanding of the benefits and costs of employment relative to financial and personal needs.

Skill Area 2: "What Type of Job Should You Apply For?" Clients are helped to decide if they have realistic vocational goals based on past work and educational experience before beginning their job searches. This skill area is not an in-depth vocational exploration exercise but rather is designed to screen people with unrealistic expectations and refer them to ancillary services before they enter the program. This practice ensures that clients have reasonable job goals before they undertake comprehensive job searches.

Skill Area 3: Locating Job Leads. Clients are next taught how to find and use job leads according to the types of work that they are seeking. Because different jobs use different types of leads, the variety of available leads can become staggering. To avoid overwhelming clients with too much information, five common job leads are covered that have been most effective in helping participants find work in the past. These include classified ads, the Yellow Pages, civil service announcements, networking, and business canvassing. In addition, ten secondary and more specialized sources of job leads, useful for specific job goals, are also presented to individual clients as needed.

Skill Area 4: Contacting Employers. How to follow up on job leads by telephone or in person is the focus of this skill area. The first section covers proper telephone technique, how to prepare for a call, points to cover when making the call, and how to turn "dead-end" calls, ones in which the positions have been filled, into sources of new information. Clients participate in a variety of discussion, workbook, and role-play exercises during the course of training. Training of in-person employer contact skills follows a similar pattern. First, clients view a videotape segment that contrasts proper and improper techniques; next, they discuss the segment and then pair off and role-play in-person contacts with an employer, thus remediating skills to proficiency.

Skill Area 5: Filling Out Job Applications. Clients next learn how to complete job applications. Although application forms vary in length, most can be dissected into seven basic sections: personal history, job preference, availability, educational history, personal abilities, work history, and references. Clients learn how to respond to these questions on any application form and how to tailor answers to specific jobs by emphasizing their relevant personal history, experience, and training. A "Truth and Ethics" section covers client responsibility to provide accurate information, what questions employers may or may not be allowed to ask, and how to handle overly intrusive questions. Clients also learn how to honestly and effectively answer "problem questions," which, if not handled carefully, can affect their opportunities for employment.

Skill Area 6: The Job Interview. In this skill area, clients practice job interviews, with attention to factors such as being appropriately groomed and dressed, arriving on time, demonstrating good social skills, and effectively answering interview questions. Clients research answers to typical job interview questions as well as practice interviews via role plays. Individual performance deficits are identified during the course of training, and specific remedial exercises are prescribed to establish consistent abilities. Because job interview performance is so critical to employment outcome, significantly more training time is spent in this skill area than in the other six areas of the job-seeking skills training curriculum.

Skill Area 7: Finalizing a Job Offer. In this last skill area, clients learn how to evaluate and finalize job offers by reviewing the terms of each offer received, weighing its merits and costs, and discussing the position with the employer. Program experience shows that most job offers are reasonable. However, some job offers are "come-ons," offering substandard pay, poor working conditions, or inadequate benefits. In other situations, a job offer is valid, but the client and employer have different understandings about the position and its compensation. Resolution of these situations requires clear communication with the employer and the ability to negotiate changes as necessary. Similar to other skill areas, discussion, workbook, and video and role-play exercises are used as training techniques in these skills.

Client Workbook

The client workbook parallels the training curriculum, providing all exercises and checklists involved with job-seeking skills training. The workbook is designed as an individualized reference instrument for each client, helping clients tailor training to their personal situations. As they fill out each exercise, clients develop critical information and material that helps them conduct their own job searches. The tasks include setting vocational goals, identifying personal and business references, developing model job application forms, coordinating educational and vocational histories, preparing for and participating in job interviews, and other relevant endeavors. This individualized approach helps each client organize a job search from the start and prospectively manage anxiety-producing and possibly detrimental situations.

Getting a Job: Job-Seeking Skills Video

The videocassette covers each of the seven skill areas of the job-seeking skills training curriculum and runs approximately fifty minutes in length. The tape is presented in segments, corresponding to the materials being trained at the time. For each skill area, the videotape models appropriate skills that clients would be expected to present during a job search, as well as issues for discussion that are germane to the question-and-answer sessions of each skill area. Thus, in Skill Area 1, the benefits and costs of employment are presented along with vignettes of people who have either carefully or haphazardly plotted out their job searches. In Skill Area 2, the right and wrong ways to look for a job are presented. A similar approach is presented for the remaining skill areas of the video.

Job Search

After completing the formal training of job-seeking skills, clients begin individualized job searches. In addition to providing a physical and social environment conducive to a job search, counselors must also structure daily activities in the program. Four areas critical to job outcomes include goal setting, the daily job search, the program's incentive system, and monitoring of clients' performance.

Goal Setting. A goal-setting group begins each day for all job seekers. Participants meet with staff to review the previous day's progress, set individual goals for the current day's job search, and trade potential job leads with other participants. Goals are individualized for each client, based on the type of job that he or she is seeking and the previous day's performance in the program. Most clients are able to manage three to four prioritized goals per day, and a typical day's list may include the activities of reviewing fresh job leads, calling back old leads, making new phone calls, filling out application forms, mailing letters, and actually interviewing for a job. Because different tasks take different amounts of time, it is important to ensure that selected goals can be completed within the program day and are relevant to the client's overall job search.

The goal-setting session is also a time when counselors can meet with clients to assess the presence of other problems that might directly interfere with the job search (for example, the need to see a psychiatrist to regulate psychotropic medication). Although the program may not be able to directly assist the client with a given problem, it can give the client the time required to address the situation or refer the client to appropriate resources, offering them the opportunity to return to the Job Finding Club when the issue has been resolved.

Daily Job Search. After the morning meeting, clients follow their structured goals throughout the day with intermittent contacts by a "floor counselor" to assess progress. This person continuously rotates among clients to monitor their progress and provide assistance for various daily problems. Counselors are also available to facilitate problem solving in novel situations, although participants are expected to try and address the problems first on their own.

Not all clients are present in the program all of the time. Some clients leave for job interviews or for program-related appointments, to canvass local businesses for jobs, and to attend to other needs. Similar to any job, clients are expected to check out with the counselor before leaving and provide an estimated time of return. The client then reports back to the counselor upon return with verification of the activities in which he or she was engaged. With few exceptions, such as a late afternoon job interview, all clients return to the program to check out before leaving at the end of the day.

Incentive System. A two-tier monetary incentive system based on participant productivity was established to further motivate client participation. This incentive system serves two purposes. First, it helps motivate client participation during prolonged and often discouraging periods of job searching. Initial attempts to use the "generic" Job Club buddy system were ineffective because many participants are socially withdrawn, have problems working on the more complex skills involved in a partnership, such as the buddy system required, or are looking for markedly different types of jobs. Second, the monetary incentive system provides often-indigent clients with funds to meet ancillary costs involved in a job search (for example, telephone calls or bus fare). The money that they earn from participation in the project is enough to meet these needs but is insufficient to live on, thereby motivating their earnest efforts toward looking for jobs rather than indefinitely staying in the program.

Monitoring Clients' Performance. A job search is an individual effort, and each client's performance must be closely monitored. The competency-based training curriculum, daily goal setting, and frequent monitoring of daily activities make it possible to keep on top of client performance and expectations with relatively short notice. In addition, formal biweekly progress reviews between individual clients and staff provide another perspective on goal attainment. When monitoring systems are closely adhered to, clients are more likely to remain on task and find employment. On the other hand, haphazard monitoring of client performance results in few positive placements. Through proper management of the feedback built into the system, it is possible to increase outcome and decrease work loads for everybody involved.

The Job-Finding Club as a Rehabilitation Technology

Our research over the past decade has identified several factors that strongly correlate to employment outcomes for persons with psychiatric disorders. These include diagnosis and severity of psychopathology, type of disability benefit received, vocational history, and job-seeking skills. These factors do not appear to be mutually exclusive and often combine to affect outcomes.

By the time a person is referred for vocational rehabilitation services, the individual's level of job-seeking skills is the only attribute available for direct intervention. The person's other characteristics are either historical or diagnostic in nature and cannot be changed. Although good job-seeking skills alone are insufficient to ensure job placement, they may help override other negative prognostics, allowing the person a chance to find a job. Thus, persons with excellent job interview skills may be able to persuade an employer that their spotty job histories are behind them and that they now can be valuable members of a firm. The organization of the Job Finding Club can help a person deficient in job search skills, but technically proficient in his or her vocation, organize a successful job search. The program can also help the individual overcome disincentives associated with disability benefits such as fear of loss of benefits or of the ability to remain employed. These issues can be addressed by helping clients secure high-paying, stable positions that are tailored to their abilities.

The Job-Finding Club as a Management System

The program can also be considered a management system that maximizes both client and professional resources. The services of teaching clients necessary job-seeking skills and providing the proper supports transfer the major effort and responsibilities to those who have the time and will directly benefit. Vocational counselors and vocational rehabilitation systems also benefit as the structure of the program directs the activities of professional staff and improves accountability. With the explicit goal of training clients in job-seeking skills to secure employment, staff can more easily focus their daily activities and avoid distractions from ancillary duties that are not related to program operations.

Perhaps the biggest challenge to any program is to contain its focus. A program that is successful in one area is often expanded to address other challenges. Sooner or later, the initially explicit and successful program expands into a nebulous system that "serves" many but helps few. By recognizing the unique and explicit goal of the Job Finding Club, however, it has been possible to maintain its direction.

Summary

The opportunity to return to work is often the culmination of extensive and collaborative efforts by clients, psychiatrists, and allied mental health and rehabilitation practitioners. Successful vocational placement and tenure is a victory not only for each individual client but also for the comprehensive set of services and supports established to foster this self-determination. Much as a chain is only as strong as its links, successful job placement must be viewed as but one link in a comprehensive rehabilitation program. Our research in competitive community employment placement over the past decade has resulted in the development of the Job Finding Module, as our contribution to one link of this evolving chain of necessary treatment and rehabilitation services for the seriously mentally ill.

References

Anthony, W. A., Buell, G. J., Sharratt, S., and Althoff, M. E. "Efficacy of Psychiatric Rehabilitation." *Psychological Bulletin,* 1972, *78,* 447–456.

Anthony, W. A., Cohen, M. R., and Vitalo, R. "The Measurement of Rehabilitation Outcome." *Schizophrenia Bulletin,* 1978, *4,* 365-383.

Anthony, W. A., and Jansen, M. A. "Predicting the Vocational Capacity of the Chronically Mentally Ill: Research and Policy Implications." *American Psychologist,* 1984, *39,* 537-544.

Azrin, N. H. *The Job-Finding Club as a Method for Obtaining Eligible Clients: Demonstration, Evaluation, and Counselor Training.* Final report, no. 51-17-76104. Washington, D.C.: U.S. Department of Labor, 1978.

Azrin, N. H., and Besalel, V. A. *Job Club Counselors Manual: A Behavioral Approach to Vocational Counseling.* Baltimore, Md.: University Park Press, 1980.

Azrin, N. H., Flores, T., and Kaplan, S. J. "Job-Finding Club: A Group Assisted Program for Obtaining Employment." *Behavior Research and Therapy,* 1975, *13,* 17-27.

Azrin, N. H., and Phillip, R. A. "The Job Club Method for the Job Handicapped: A Comparative Outcome Study." *Rehabilitation Counseling Bulletin,* 1979, *23,* 144-155.

Jacobs, H. E. "Vocational Rehabilitation." In R. P. Liberman (ed.), *Psychiatric Rehabilitation of Chronic Mental Patients.* Washington, D.C.: American Psychiatric Press, 1988.

Jacobs, H. E., Collier, R., Wissusik, D., Stackman, D., and Burkeman, D. "The Brentwood Job Finding Club: Correlates of Vocational Outcome for the Psychiatrically Disabled." Unpublished manuscript, Department of Psychiatry, University of California, Los Angeles, 1991.

Jacobs, H. E., Donahoe, C. P., and Falloon, I.R.H. "Rehabilitation of the Chronic Schizophrenic." In E. Pan, S. Newman, T. Backer, and C. Vash (eds.), *Annual Review of Rehabilitation.* Vol. 4. New York: Springer, 1985.

Jacobs, H. E., Kardashian, S., Kreinbring, R. K., Ponder, R., and Simpson, A. R. "A Skills-Oriented Model for Facilitating Employment Among Psychiatrically Disabled Persons." *Rehabilitation Counseling Bulletin,* 1984, *28,* 87-96.

Mitchell, J., Jacobs, H. E., and Yen, F. "Costs and Response Rates in a Community Follow-up for a Psychiatric Vocational Rehabilitation Program." *Rehabilitation Counseling Bulletin,* 1987, *31,* 273-277.

HARVEY E. JACOBS, Ph.D., is a research psychologist at the Drucker Brain Injury Center, Moss Rehabilitation Hospital, Philadelphia. He directed the design and implementation of the Job-Finding Club program and is author of the Job-Finding Module.

ROSEMARY COLLIER, M.S., is staff research associate, Department of Psychiatry and Biobehavioral Sciences, UCLA School of Medicine. She coordinated the Job-Finding Club research program and the development of the Job-Finding Module.

DONALD WISSUSIK, M.A., C.R.C., is clinical supervisor, Springbrook Institute, Newberg, Oregon. He served as chief vocational rehabilitation counselor for the Job-Finding Club program during its development and evaluation in the Rehabilitation Medicine Service of the Brentwood (Psychiatric) Division of the West Los Angeles VA Medical Center.

INDEX

Achievement-linked attributions, 15–16
Affect-linked attributions, 14–15
Ague, C., 81, 84
Allness, D. J., 34, 40
Alumni meetings, program, 101–102
Ambulatory aftercare, 80
Anderson, C. M., 47, 48, 51, 83, 84
Angrist, B., 67, 76
Anthony, W. A., 87, 88, 89, 90, 91, 92, 95, 96, 99, 103
Antipsychotic medication, 24, 70–71, 76
Applications, job, 110
Art therapy, 25–26
Asarnow, R. F., 71, 76
Assessment, 38–39; continuous ecobehavioral, 82–83; CRU program, 68–69, 70–71; DDTP programs, 58; interviews of patients, 22–23, 47, 89–90, 94; of patients and therapists, 36. See also Case studies
Atkinson, R. M., 57, 63
Attributional processes, 14–16
Ayllon, T., 61, 62
Azrin, N. H., 61, 62, 74, 77, 106, 115

Baccus, M., 88, 96
Bachrach, L. L., 59, 63
Baldessarini, R. J., 70, 76
Beck, A. T., 14, 18
Behavior therapy: cognitive, 10–11, 21–22, 31; CRU program, 68–71, 72–75
Behavioral Family Management. See Psychoeducational (PE) multifamily groups
Beliefs: attributional, 14–16; identification of, 25, 72
Benefit-risk ratio, neuroleptic dosage, 3, 70–71, 72
Berman, K. F., 12–13, 19
Besalel, V. A., 106, 115
Biosocial Treatment Research Division (New York), 44
Bipolar affective disorder, 12, 101–102
Blackwell, G., 42
Blanch, A. K., 87, 95
Bond, G. R., 81, 84, 87, 92, 95
Boston University Center for Psychiatric Rehabilitation, 4, 88–93

Bowen, L., 3, 78
Bowers, M. B., 57, 63
BPRS, 36, 70
Brain-storming, group, 49–50
Brenner, H. D., 16–17, 18, 68, 76
Brentwood VA Medical Center, 34–38, 57–62, 62, 68; Job-Finding Club, 107–114. See also UCLA
Brentwood Veterans Affairs Medical Center, 4, 97–99, 102–103
Brief Psychiatric Rating Scale (BPRS), 36, 70
Brooke, V., 88, 96
Buddy system, Job Club, 113

Camarillo State Hospital. See Clinical Research Unit (CRU)
Carey, K. B., 61, 63
Case management, 91, 113, 114; defining, 40; expansion of, 33–34, 91–92, 101; FACT program, 44–51; and social skills training, 34, 35, 36–37, 38–39, 79–80; TCL and PACT, 59–60
Case studies, 11, 13–14, 15–16, 37–38; choose-get-keep, 93–95; CRU, 71–75; DDTP, 59–62; dialogues, 22–23, 26–27, 28–29; ecological vocational rehabilitation, 79–80; FACT, 50–51; optimal drug therapy, 71–75; Veterans' garden, 97–98, 100–101, 101–102. See also Patients, mental
Cheadle, A. J., 81, 85
Choose-get-keep rehabilitation approach, 4, 88–95, 99
Ciompi, L., 81, 84
Cipani, E., 76
Classes. See Training
Client workbooks, 111
Clinical deterioration, 70–71
Clinical Global Impressions Scale scores, 70, 71
Clinical Research Unit (CRU), Camarillo-UCLA, 3, 68–71
Coaching. See Job-coaching
Cocaine abuse, 55, 60–61
Cognition impairments, 7–8
Cognitive therapy viewpoint, 25, 26

Cognitive-behavioral treatment program components, 24-30
Cohen, B. F., 89, 96
Cohen, B. M., 70, 76
Cohen, M. R., 89, 91, 95, 96
Collaborative empiricism, 25
Collier, R., 108, 115
Community members, support of, 47, 91-92
Community-based treatment, 2-3, 44-51, 93
Computerized task exercises, 9
Concept formation and processing, 12-14
Contingency management, 15-16
Continuity, case management, 59-60
Continuous performance impairments, 8-10
Contracts, patient-therapy program, 23-24, 50
Coping skills, 60
Corrigan, P. W., 36, 41
Costs of therapy programs, 5, 31, 93
Cousino, I., 104
Credit incentive program, DDTP, 61-62
Crisis intervention, 46, 83
Criteria, patient's job, 89-90, 94
CRU. See Clinical Research Unit (CRU)

Danley, K. S., 88, 90, 92, 95, 96, 98, 103
Dauwalder, J. P., 4, 81, 84
DDTP. See Dual Diagnosis Treatment Program (DDTP)
Deinstitutionalization, 33, 43, 55
Delusions, misperception, 72, 74
Denudativeness, 72
Depression, post-program, 40
DeRisi, W. J., 17, 18
Disclosure, mental disability, 91
Disorientation, treatment of, 12
Distortions, cognitive, 28, 30
Distractibility, 10-11
Dixon, L., 56, 63
Documentation, patient's job search: 36-37, 111. See also Manuals, training
Donahoe, C. P., 106, 115
Donnelan, A. M., 76, 77
Dosage, optimal antipsychotic: 3, 70-71, 76. See also Medication
Drug abuse by schizophrenics, 55-62
Drug subculture, 56

Dual Diagnosis Treatment Program (DDTP), 57-62

Earnings, program participant, 92, 113
Eating program, 69
Eckman, T. A., 65
Ecological vocational rehabilitation, 79-83
Education: co-worker, 82-83; family, 47-48; in vivo, 46, 60, 82; vocational training, 82-83, 101
Emotional states, cognition of, 27-28
Employers, cooperation with, 81, 82-83, 91-92, 110
Employment: choose-get-keep supported, 88-93; ecological support of, 79-83; Job Club support of, 99, 106, 106-109, 113; outcomes, 46, 81, 92-93; patient's history of, 47, 89, 93, 99, 108; PE multifamily group support of, 49-50. See also Vocational rehabilitation
Employment Support Services (Boston), 88-95
Engagement sessions, 47
Engel, J. D., 36, 41
England, experiment in Buckinghamshire, 5
Environment, ecobehavioral, 79-83
Epidemiological studies, 55
Evaluation, patient, 35, 36, 99; ongoing, 30; problem-focused, 22-23. See also Case management
Evaluation, program. See Assessment
Extinction of attention, 69

FACT. See Family-Aided Assertive Community Treatment (FACT)
Falloon, I.R.H., 5, 6, 48, 52, 106, 115
Family involvement in therapy, 4, 12, 24, 30, 44, 45-51, 80, 83
Family-Aided Assertive Community Treatment (FACT), 45-51
Farkas, M. D., 88, 91, 95
Farrelly, F., 44, 52
Flores, T., 106, 115
Focus, containment of program, 114
Friel, T. W., 89, 96

Generalization skills, 36
Glynn, S. M., 1, 6
Goal setting by patients: cognitive-behavioral program, 23; independent

living skills, 34-35, 39; PE multifamily group and, 47-48, 49; social, 17; vocational, 37, 49, 88-90, 99, 107, 109-110, 112, 113
Gold, M. S., 57, 63
Goodrich, V., 10, 11, 13, 18
Gordon, J. R., 59, 63
Granovetter, M. S., 49, 52
Grodall, P., 88, 96
Group: cognitive-behavioral therapy, 25-28; daily goal-setting, 112; DDTP treatment schedule, 58; discussion of emotional states, 27-28; PE multifamily, 44, 47-50; therapy, 25-28, 57; training in social skills, 100-101

Hagner, J., 89, 96
Hallucination, control over, 28-29
Haloperidol (Haldol) dosage, 70-71, 76
Harris, M., 59, 63
Hellerstein, D., 57, 63
Hierholzer, R. W., 100, 103
Hiett, A., 49, 53
History, patient's employment, 47, 89, 93, 108
Hodel, B., 16-17, 18
Hoffmann, H., 4, 80, 84
Hogarty, G. E., 39, 41, 47, 48, 51, 83, 84
Homelessness, 55, 60-61, 62
Homework, patient, 30
Honingfeld, G., 68, 77
Horticulture therapy, 4, 99-103
Hygiene, personal, 62, 69, 72

In vivo therapy. See Milieu therapy
Incentive system, 73; achievement-linked attribution, 15-16; CRU credit, 69; DDTP credit card, 61-62; identification of, 35; job searching, 113; monetary, 113. See also Motivation factors
Independence and the family attachment, 30
Independent Living Skills Survey, 35
Individual therapy, 10, 17, 36-37; sessions, 28-29, 73-76
Individualized Written Rehabilitation Plans, 36-37
Instruction, competency-based, 36
Interventions: job-coaching, 4, 94-95, 97-98, 101-102, 112-113; job-seeking skills, 113-114; milieu therapy, 24-25,

46; optimal drug and behavior therapy, 70-71, 72-75; PACT, 33-34, 44, 46, 59; PE multifamily group, 47-51; research on effectiveness of, 75-76, 103; TCL, 44-46
Interviews: board-and-care home, 37-38; cognitive therapy, 28-29; job, 94, 110-111; patient assessment, 22-23, 47, 89-90, 94
Intolerable behaviors, treatment of, 69-71

Jacobs, H. E., 106, 107, 108, 115
Job Club employment support programs, 5, 99, 106, 106-109, 113
Job finding, individualized, 36-37, 49-50, 83, 99; choose-get-keep approach to, 88-95
Job losses, 92-93, 102
Job search activities, 49-50, 88-90, 112-113
Job-coaching, 4, 94-95, 97-98, 101-102, 112-113
Job-Finding Module, 4, 105-106; outcomes, 107-108, 113-114; search activities, 112-113; skill areas, 109-111; training manuals, 108-109
Jobs, competitive, employment in, 83, 88-95, 110

Kane, J., 68, 77
Kania, J., 57, 63
Kaplan, S. J., 106, 115
Knoedler, W. H., 34, 40
Kofoed, L., 57, 63
Kraemer, S., 8, 18
Krekorian, H.A.R., 5, 6
Kube, G., 16-17, 18
Kuehnel, T. G., 78

Laporta, M., 5, 6
LaVigna, G. W., 76, 77
Leads, job, 110
Lehman Quality of Life Scale, 39
Lentz, R., 76, 77
Liaison, psychiatric team—general practitioner, 5
Liberman, R. P., 1, 6, 8, 17, 18, 34, 35, 36, 37, 41, 42, 48, 52, 58, 59, 64, 76, 77, 78, 99, 100, 103
Los Angeles, University of California at. See UCLA

Los Angeles VA Medical Center, West, 55, 57
Ludwig, A. M., 44, 52
Lukoff, D., 35, 52

McCrory, D., 90, 96
MacDonald-Wilson, K. L., 88, 90, 92, 96
Mancuso, L. L., 88, 90, 92, 96
Manuals, training, 26, 108-109
Marder, S. R., 36, 41, 70, 77
Marlatt, G. A., 59, 63
Marshall, B. D., Jr., 78
Matching, job, 90-91
Medication, 40; drug abuse and, 56; reduced dosages of antipsychotic, 24, 70-71; refractoriness to, 67-68, 70; self-management of, 15, 24, 36, 50-51, 59
Meehan, B., 57, 63
Meltzer, H. Y., 68, 77
Milieu therapy, 24-25, 46; multifamily group, 48-49
Miller, S., 48, 53
Minkoff, K., 58, 63
Mitchell, J., 108, 115
Modeling, job-search skills, 111-112
Molecular cognition functions, 7-8, 12, 16-17
Moller, H., 8, 18
Money management skills, 60, 94-95
Monitoring. See Case management
Moon, S., 88, 96
Morgan, R., 81, 85
Motivation factors: 9-10, 17, 26, 28. See also Incentive system; Self-management
Mueser, R. T., 17, 18
Mueser, T. I., 1, 6
Multidimensional model for psychiatric rehabilitation, 99
Multidisciplinary programs. See Team approach

Nebraska Psychiatric Institute, 3
Networks: multi-family, 47-48, 49, 51; sociopsychiatric, 79-83
Neuroleptic drug therapy, 70-76
New York State Psychiatric Institute, 44
Nisbet, J., 89, 96
Novas, D. B., 98, 103
Nuechterlein, K. H., 8, 18, 35, 52
Nurse therapists, 21, 31

Occupational therapy, psychosocial, 38-39
Offers, evaluating job, 111
Oltmanns, T. F., 10, 18
Optimization, neuroleptic drug therapy, 70-71, 76; case study, 71-75
Orientation and self-monitoring, 12, 16
Outpatient treatment for schizophrenic substance abusers, 57, 61

PACT. See Program of Assertive Community Treatment (PACT)
Paranoid schizophrenia. See Schizophrenia
Patients, mental, 1-2; choose-get-keep activities of, 88-95; ecological environment of, 79-83; employment history, 47, 89, 93, 99, 108; quality of life, 39, 75-76; relapse by, 39, 45-46, 48, 59, 60-61, 71; selection of for programs, 21-22, 27-28, 45, 67-68, 81, 82, 88. See also Case studies; Self-management
Paul, G. L., 76, 77
PE. See Psychoeducational (PE) multifamily groups
Penn, D. L., 8, 18, 20
Period of therapy contract, 23-24
Perris, C., 3, 32
Pet animal therapy, 24
Pharmacotherapy, behavior therapy and, 3, 68, 70-71, 76
Phillip, R. A., 106, 115
Pia, D., 80, 84
Pierce, R. M., 89, 96
Pitts, D. B., 34, 41, 98, 103
"Place-then-train" vocational rehabilitation, 87-88, 89, 97-98
Placement activities, 90-92
Pogue-Geile, M. F., 10, 18
Post, R. M., 57, 63
Post-traumatic stress disorder (PTSD), 98
Primary care practitioners, 5
Principles, cognitive therapy, 25
Private-sector participation. See Employers; Employment
Problem inventory, patient, 22, 73, 76
Problem-solving skills, patient, 46, 60
Prognosis for stimulant-abusing schizophrenic patients, 56-57
Program of Assertive Community Treatment (PACT), 33-34, 44, 46, 59

Protective factors, role of, 1-2
Psychoeducational (PE) multifamily groups, 44, 47-50
Psychopharmacological treatment, 35-36
Psychosocial treatment of schizophrenia, 44-51, 58
PTSD, 98

Quality of life, patient, 39, 75-76
Questions: cognitive training, 26-27; training in handling, 110; written rehabilitation plan, 37

Rating instruments, 11, 30, 36, 39, 70, 71
Readiness, job, 109
Reed, D., 3, 9, 20
Rehabilitation: cognitive impairments and, 7-8; CRU program, 69; FACT program, 46-51. See also Vocational rehabilitation
Rehabilitation Act of 1986, 91-92
Reinforcement, differential, 73
Reiss, D. J., 47, 48, 51
Relapse, patient, 39, 45-46, 48, 71; prevention training, 59, 60-61
Relationship, collaborative empirical, 25
Relaxation therapy, 73, 74
Residual cognitive impairments, 7-8
Resources, management of professional, 114
Response cost procedure, 69
Responsibilities, increasing patient, 47, 89
Rituals, compulsive, 15-16
Roberts, L. J., 4, 64
Roessler, R. T., 49, 53
Rogers, E. S., 98, 103
Round table drop-in facility, 80

Schizophrenia: cognitive behavior therapy and, 10-11, 21-22, 31; conceptual impairments and, 12-13; concomitant stimulant-abuse and, 55-57; FACT and TCL treatment of, 45-46; family bond and, 44, 47-50; neuroleptic drug treatment of, 70-71, 72-75; psychosocial treatment of, 44-51, 58. See also Case studies
Schulz, S. C., 67, 76
Sciarappa, K., 96
Screaming, episodic, 72-73

Section 504C. See Rehabilitation Act of 1986
Self-esteem by patients, 15, 26, 28
Self-help firms for former patients, 81
Self-management: behavioral, 58-59, 60, 73, 76; of medication, 15, 24, 36, 50-51, 59; of symptoms, 59, 60, 61, 74-75
Self-monitoring, cognitive function of, 12, 16
Service coordination, 5, 91, 93, 101
Seyfried, E., 81, 85
Shanahan, W., 5, 6
Shaner, A., 64
Short-term memory skills, 11, 12
Side effects, antipsychotic medication, 70-71
Significant others, employment support by, 90. See also Family involvement in therapy
Singer, J., 68, 77
Singularity of impairments, 10, 17
Skill areas. See Social skills; Vocational rehabilitation
Social and Independent Living Skills Program, 34-38; empirical evaluation, 38-39
Social apperception exercises, 11, 13
Social cognition and role performance, 16-17
Social Security, 4, 95; Disability Insurance (SSDI), 108
Social skills: training technologies, 8, 16-17, 26, 33-34, 36, 58-59, 60, 74, 79-83, 100-101; for the workplace, 79-83, 98, 100-101, 109-111. See also Self-management
Span of Apprehension Test, 71
Spaulding, W., 8, 11, 13, 18, 20
Spohn, H., 7, 18
SSDI and SSI beneficiaries, 108
Stamina assessment, 99
Statistics: choose-get-keep program, 92-93; job-finding, 4-5, 81, 107-108; therapy program, 30, 57
Stein, L. I., 33-34, 40, 41, 59, 64
Stimulant abuse by schizophrenics, 55-62
Storms, L., 10, 11, 13, 18
Strachan, A., 44, 53
Strauss, M., 7, 18
"Stress-vulnerability" model of illness, 1-2, 57, 58

Stuve, P., 20
Subsistence competencies, 105, 108
Successful Living format, 100
Sullivan, M., 10, 11, 13, 18, 20
Supplemental Security Income (SSI), 108
Supported employment, 4, 97–98
Sweden, University of Umea, 3, 21, 31
Switzerland, ecological vocational program in, 4, 79–86
Symptom management training, 59, 60, 61, 74–75
Symptom-linked attributions, treatment of, 14–15

TCL. See Training in Community Living (TCL)
Team approach, 5; CRU program, 68; ·DDTP program, 57–58; ecological vocational rehabilitation, 81–83; TCL program, 47, 59
Teicher, M. H., 70, 76
Test, M. A., 33–34, 34, 40, 41, 44, 53, 59, 64
Thematic apperception test (TAT) cards, 11
Therapeutic window, medication plasma levels, 3, 71
Time-out from positive reinforcement, 69
Torrey, E. F., 59, 64
Training: behavioral self-management skills, 58–59, 60; cognitive-behavioral, 26–27, 28–29; in conceptual processing, 12–14, 25; in continuous performance, 8–10; ecological vocational, 79–83; formal class, 36, 40, 101; group, 100–101; job search skills, 108–111; money management, 60, 94–95; social cognition, 16–17; social skills, 36, 40, 58–59, 79–80; in symptom management, 59, 60, 61, 74–75. See also Vocational rehabilitation
Training in Community Living (TCL): family involvement with, 44–46; PACT and, 33–34, 44, 46, 59; program components, 46–47
Training manuals, 26, 108–109
Training technology: social skills, 8
Treatment contract, patient, 22–24
Treatment refractoriness, 67–68
Trigger events, identifying, 73, 76
Trusted persons, 24

Tucker, D. E., 65
Turf wars, medical profession, 5
Twelve-step groups, 4, 58

UCLA, 36, 101; Camarillo-UCLA Clinical Research Unit, 3, 68–71; Clinical Research Center, 59; Department of Psychiatry, 57. See also Brentwood VA Medical Center
Unemployment rates, 81, 108
University of California, Los Angeles. See UCLA

Vaccaro, J. V., 34, 35, 37, 41, 42, 58, 59, 64, 65, 98, 103, 104
Van Putten, T., 36, 41, 70, 71, 77
Vandergoot, D. V., 49, 53
Vatcher, R., 104
Ventura, J., 35, 52
Veterans' Garden program, 4, 97–99, 102–103; components, 99–102
Video: job-seeking skills, 111–112; on schizophrenia, 48; therapy recording, 23, 30
Vietnam veterans, 97–98
Vigilance impairments, 8–10
Vitalo, R. L., 91, 95
Vocational history, patient's, 47, 89, 93, 99, 108
Vocational rehabilitation, 36–37, 45, 50–51, 81–83; choose-get-keep approach to, 88–95; competencies and prerequisites for, 82, 105–106; successfulness of, 87–88, 92–93, 107–108, 113–114. See also Employment

Wallace, C. J., 8, 18, 34, 35, 41, 42, 98, 103
Walsh, T., 57, 63
Webster, D. R., 74, 77
Weiler, M., 8, 18
Weinberger, D. R., 12–13, 19
West Los Angeles VA Medical Center, 55, 57
Willis, T. J., 76, 77
Wissusik, D., 108, 115
Wong, S. E., 76, 77
Work skills, patient. See Vocational rehabilitation
Workbook, client's job-search, 111
Workplace accommodations, reasonable, 91–92, 94

Written Rehabilitation Plans, Individualized, 36-37

Yen, F., 108, 115

Zec, R. F., 12-13, 19
Zinner, H., 8, 18

ORDERING INFORMATION

NEW DIRECTIONS FOR MENTAL HEALTH SERVICES is a series of paperback books that presents timely and readable volumes on subjects of concern to clinicians, administrators, and others involved in the care of the mentally disabled. Each volume is devoted to one topic and includes a broad range of authoritative articles written by noted specialists in the field. Books in the series are published quarterly in Fall, Winter, Spring, and Summer and are available for purchase by subscription as well as by single copy.

SUBSCRIPTIONS for 1992 cost $52.00 for individuals (a savings of 20 percent over single-copy prices) and $70.00 for institutions, agencies, and libraries. Please do not send institutional checks for personal subscriptions. Standing orders are accepted.

SINGLE COPIES cost $17.95 when payment accompanies order. (California, New Jersey, New York, and Washington, D.C., residents please include appropriate sales tax.) Billed orders will be charged postage and handling.

DISCOUNTS FOR QUANTITY ORDERS are available. Please write to the address below for information.

ALL ORDERS must include either the name of an individual or an official purchase order number. Please submit your order as follows:
  Subscriptions: specify series and year subscription is to begin
  Single copies: include individual title code (such as MHS1)

MAIL ALL ORDERS TO:
  Jossey-Bass Publishers
  350 Sansome Street
  San Francisco, California 94104

FOR SALES OUTSIDE OF THE UNITED STATES CONTACT:
  Maxwell Macmillan International Publishing Group
  866 Third Avenue
  New York, New York 10022

OTHER TITLES AVAILABLE IN THE
NEW DIRECTIONS FOR MENTAL HEALTH SERVICES SERIES
H. Richard Lamb, Editor-in-Chief

MHS52 Psychiatric Outreach to the Mentally Ill, *Neal L. Cohen*
MHS51 Treating Victims of Child Sexual Abuse, *John Briere*
MHS50 Dual Diagnosis of Major Mental Illness and Substance Disorder,
       Kenneth Minkoff, Robert Drake
MHS49 Administrative Issues in Public Mental Health, *Stuart L. Keill*
MHS48 Psychiatric Aspects of AIDS and HIV Infection, *Stephen M. Goldfinger*
MHS47 Treating Personality Disorders, *David A. Adler*
MHS46 Using Psychodynamic Principles in Public Mental Health,
       Terry A. Kupers
MHS45 New Developments in Psychiatric Rehabilitation, *Arthur T. Meyerson,
       Phyllis Solomon*
MHS44 State-University Collaboration: The Oregon Experience,
       Joseph D. Bloom
MHS43 Paying for Services: Promises and Pitfalls of Capitation,
       David Mechanic, Linda H. Aiken
MHS42 Survival Strategies for Public Psychiatry, *C. Christian Beels,
       Leona L. Bachrach*
MHS41 Legal Implications of Hospital Policies and Practices,
       Robert D. Miller
MHS40 Clinical Case Management, *Maxine Harris, Leona L. Bachrach*
MHS39 Serving the Chronically Mentally Ill in an Urban Setting:
       The Massachusetts Mental Health Center Experience, *Miles F. Shore,
       Jon E. Gudeman*
MHS38 Differing Approaches to Partial Hospitalization, *Kenneth Goldberg*
MHS37 The Perspective of John Talbott, *John A. Talbott*
MHS36 Improving Mental Health Services: What the Social Sciences
       Can Tell Us, *David Mechanic*
MHS35 Leona Bachrach Speaks: Selected Speeches and Lectures,
       Leona L. Bachrach
MHS34 Families of the Mentally Ill: Meeting the Challenges,
       Agnes B. Hatfield
MHS32 Treating Anxiety Disorders, *Rodrigo A. Muñoz*
MHS31 Eating Disorders, *Félix E. F. Larocca*
MHS29 The Elderly and Chronic Mental Illness, *Nancy S. Abramson,
       Jean K. Quam, Mona Wasow*
MHS22 Patterns of Adolescent Self-Image, *Daniel Offer, Eric Ostrov,
       Kenneth I. Howard*
MHS14 The Young Adult Chronic Patient, *Bert Pepper, Hilary Ryglewicz*